DASH DIET 2021

DASH DIET FOR BEGINNERS BOOK WITH 21 DAY MEAL PLAN

AMZ PUBLISHING

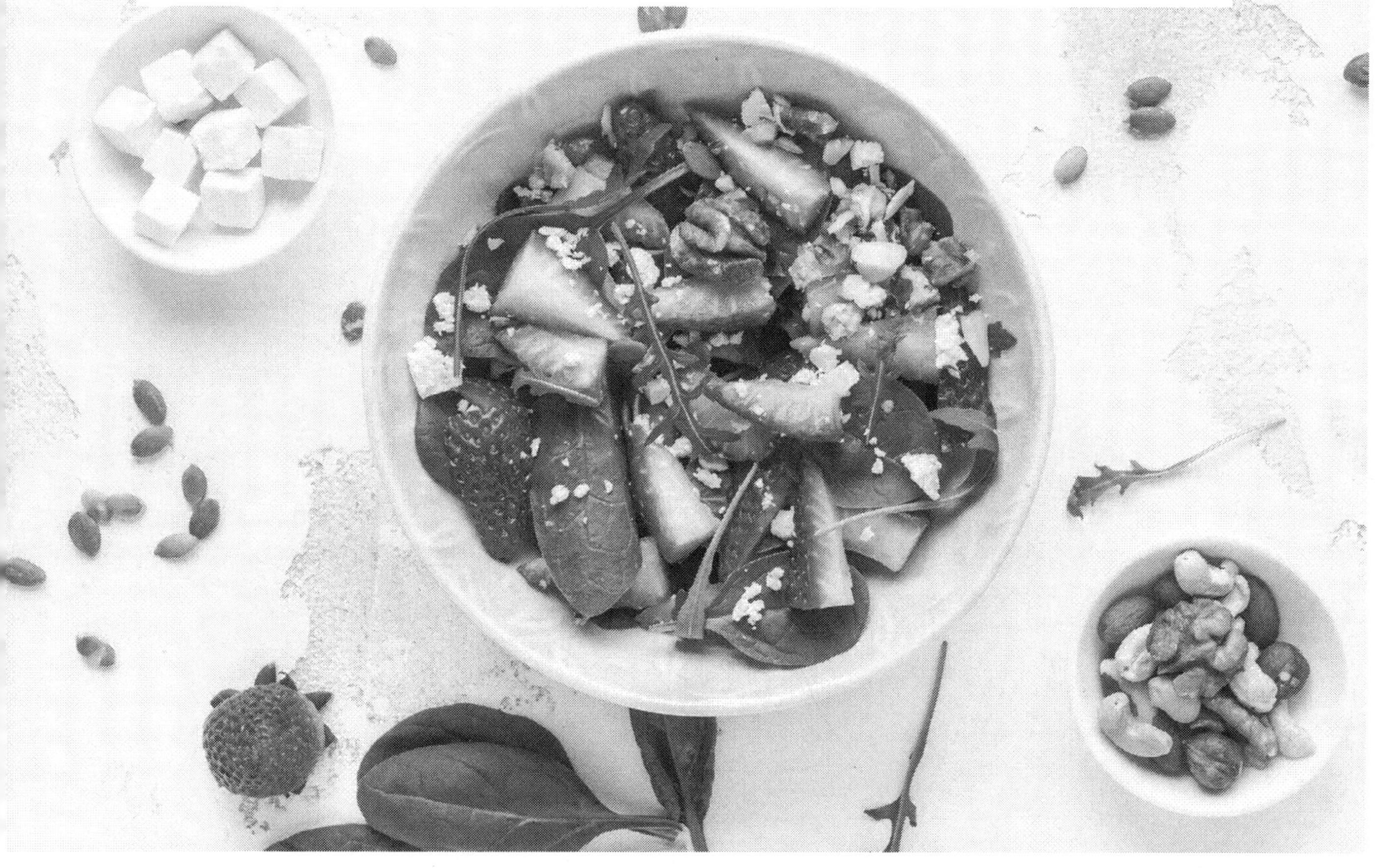

TABLE OF CONTENTS

INTRODUCTION — 4

What is Dash Diet? — 5

Benefits of Dash Diet? — 8

21-DAYS MEAL PLAN — 12

BREAKFAST RECIPES — 16

Banana And Oatmeal Pancakes — 17

Blueberry Pancakes (Whole-wheat) — 20

Breakfast Muesli Bars — 22

Cinnamon And Nutmeg French Toast — 24

Cream Cheese And Strawberry Crepes — 26

Fresh Mixed Fruit Smoothie — 28

Green Smoothie — 29

Healthy Baked Oatmeal — 30

Healthy Buckwheat Pancakes — 32

High-calorie Breakfast Smoothie — 34

Multi-grain Hot Cereal — 36

Mushroom Spinach Frittata — 38

Orange Vanilla Smoothie — 41

Overnight Refrigerated Oatmeal — 42

Overnight Refrigerated Oatmeal — 44

LUNCH RECIPES — 47

Asian-style Pork Tenderloin — 48

Baked Chicken With Herbed Wild Rice — 50

Baked Cod Topped With Capers And Lemon — 52

Baked Red Sauce Macaroni — 54

Baked Salmon Topped With Asian Marinade — 56

Brussels Sprouts With Lemon And Shallots — 58

Chicken Burritos — 60

Chicken Salad (Grilled) With Buttermilk Dressing — 62

Chicken Salad With Balsamic Vinaigrette & Pineapple — 64

TABLE OF CONTENTS

Clams Fettuccine	66
Classic Chicken Quesadillas	68
Creamy Polenta With Veggies	70
Flank Steak And Roasted Corn Salad	72
Pork Tenderloin Curry In Apple Cider	76
Strip Steak With Mushroom Whiskey Sauce	78

Dinner Recipes — 80

Asian-style Grilled Salmon	81
Baked Herb-crusted Cod	84
Barley And Tomato Roast Risotto	86
Black-eyed Creole-style Peas	90
Chicken Asparagus Penne	92
Easy Beef Brisket	94
Easy Beef Stroganoff	96
Garlic And Broccoli Rigatoni	98
Spiced Chipotle Shrimp	100
Pork Medallions In Five Spices	102
Puttanesca Served With Brown Rice	104
Roast Balsamic Chicken	106
Southwestern-style Vegan Bowl	108
Vegetarian Tofu Chili	110
White Broiled Sea Bass	112

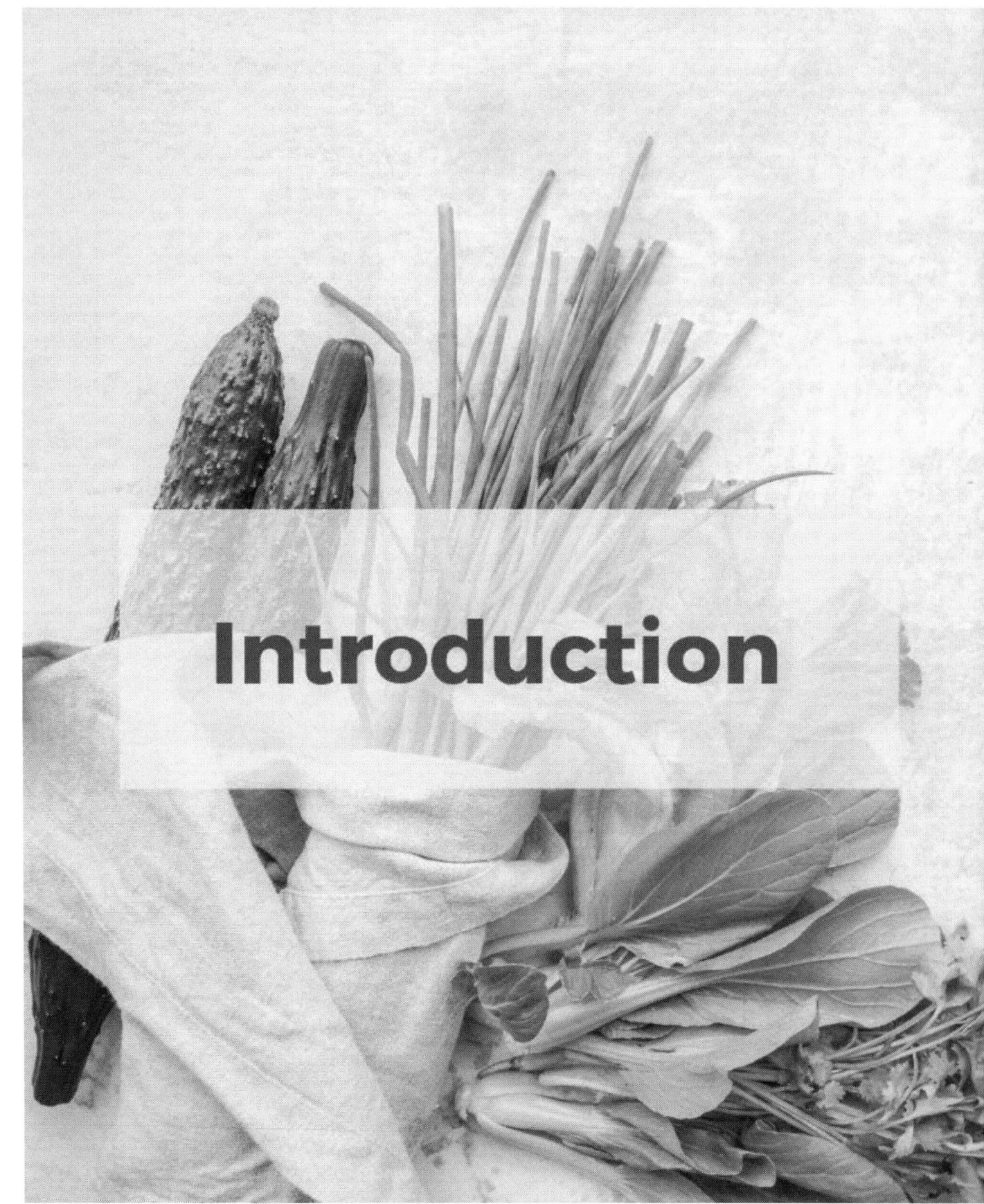

Introduction

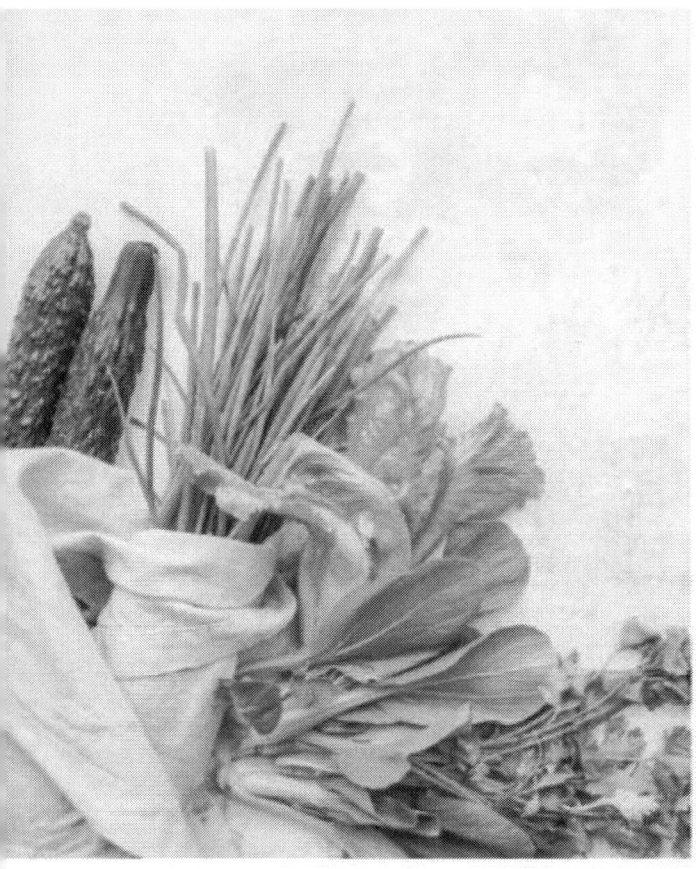
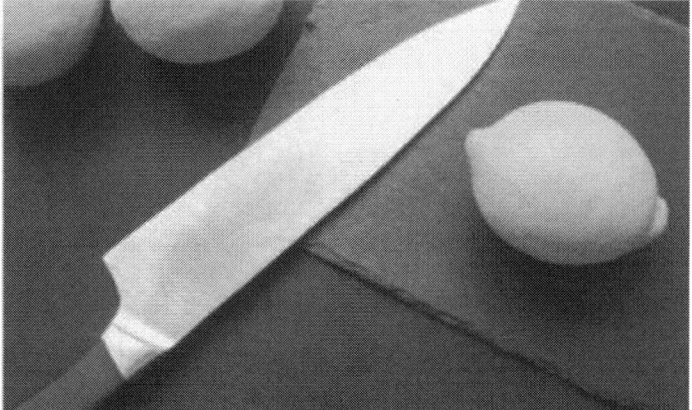
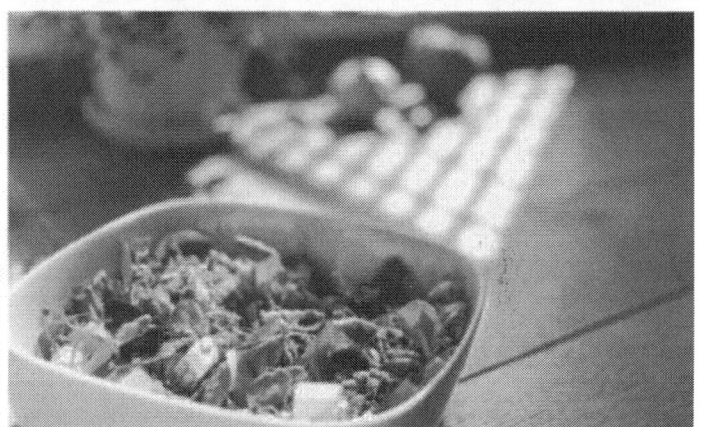

What is the DASH Diet?

With more people suffering from conditions related to high blood pressure, the DASH diet offers a unique solution that is both scientifically- and results-proven. The last decade has seen a major rise in cases related to high blood pressure with over a billion people worldwide dealing with conditions pertaining to blood pressure levels.

This constant rise has made the DASH diet one of the most effective ways to deal with this situation.

Endorsed by the United States National Heart, Lung, and Blood Institute, the DASH (Dietary Approaches to Stop Hypertension) diet studies the nutrient composition of food items to prepare unique dietary strategies that help to reduce high blood pressure.

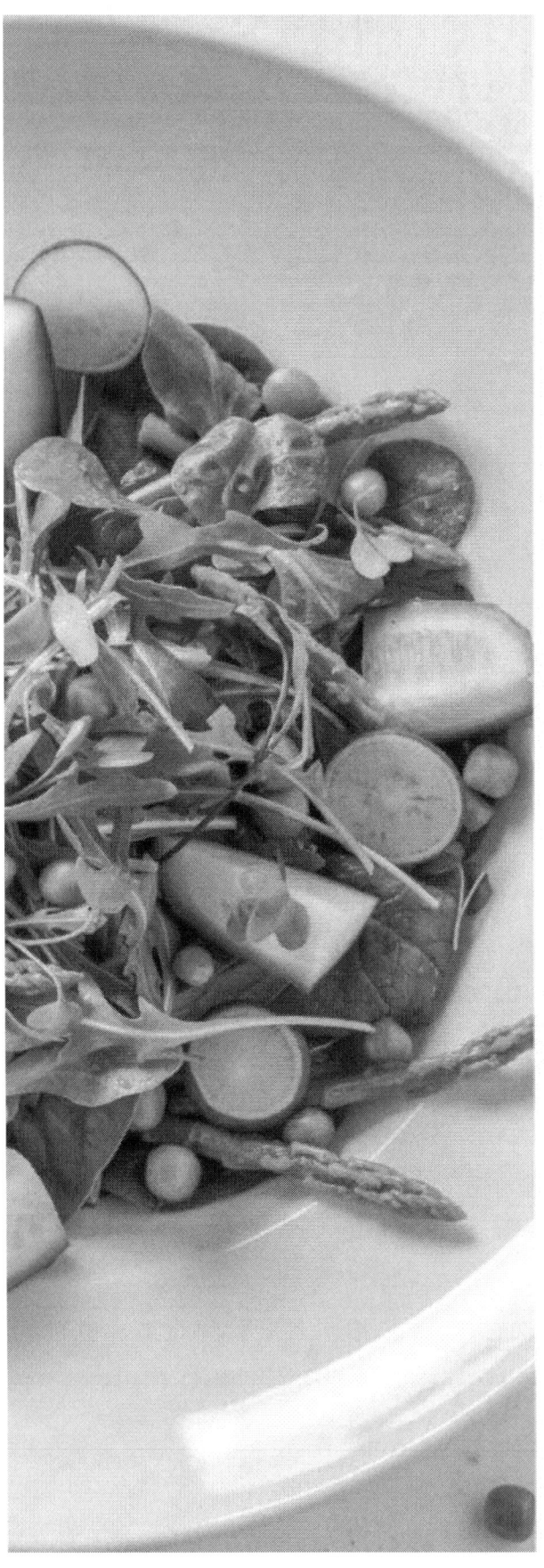

The diet is a result of the engineering done by bio-scientists and lawmakers to find the components that must be eliminated from one's diet to control the rise of blood pressure.

The DASH diet came about because the number of people complaining of high blood pressure almost doubled in the last two decades. This led medical experts, along with the United States Department of Health and Human Services, to find ways to deal with hypertension and eliminate the various risks that are associated with high blood pressure.

After a careful study, the researchers found that people who prefer to consume more vegetables or who followed a plant-based diet showed fewer signs and cases of rising blood pressure. This, therefore, became the foundation of the DASH diet.

In the DASH diet, the person focuses on consuming foods that are non-processed and more organic. Whole grains, fruits, vegetables, and lean meats form the essential components of this diet technique. In extreme cases, the person showing major signs of heart-related ailments due to high blood pressure is also advised to go vegan for some time to lower issues related to hypertension.

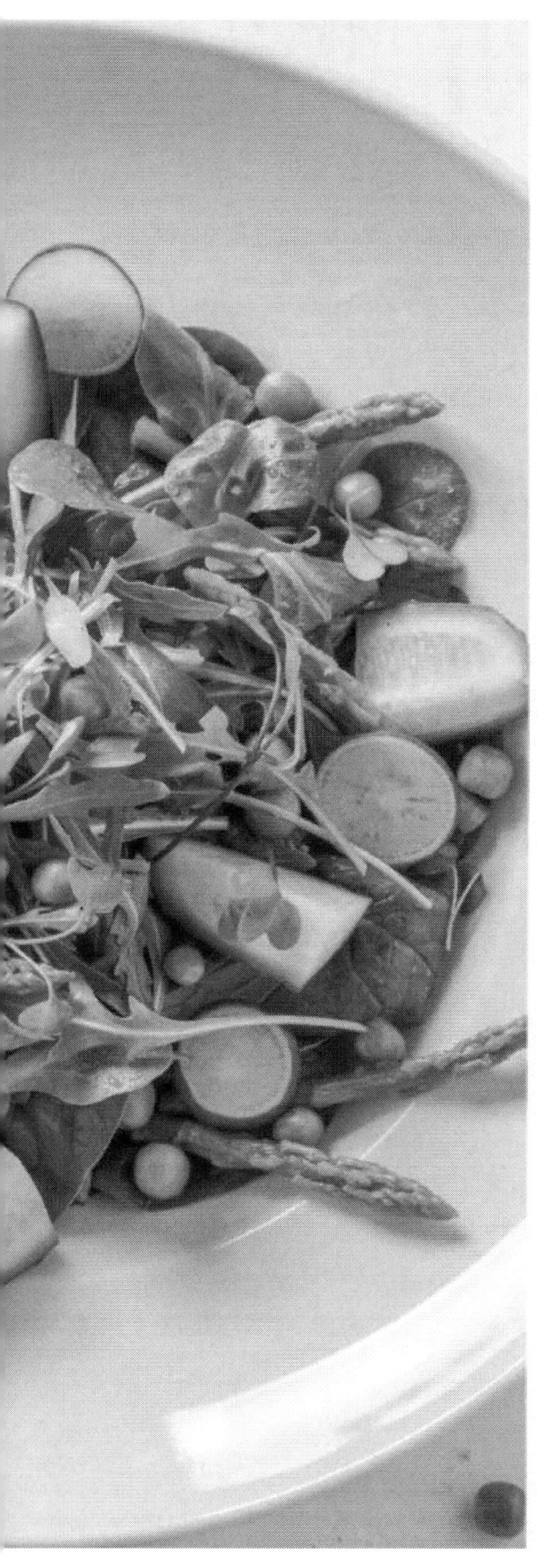

The diet also follows a strict method of using salt. Because too much salt and oil significantly raise the blood pressure in the human body, the dietary guidelines of the DASH diet significantly reduce the intake of salt.

The recipes in the DASH diet are a wholesome mix of green vegetables, natural fruits, low-fat dairy foods, and lean protein such as chicken, fish, and a lot of beans.

Besides limiting the intake of salt, the rule of thumb is to minimize food items rich in red meat, processed sugars, and composite fat.

As per the standard practice, anyone following the DASH diet is advised to not consume more than 1 teaspoon (2,300 mg) of sodium in a day.

The diet is safe to follow and is also accredited by the United States Department of Agriculture (USDA).

The US Dietary Guidelines also included the DASH diet as one of three healthy diets recommended in 2015-2020.

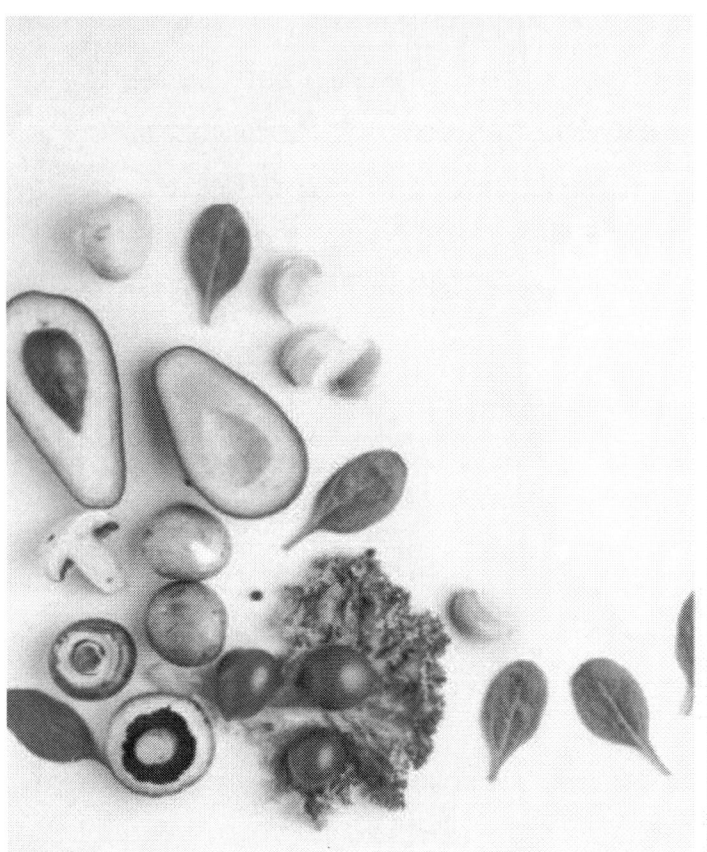
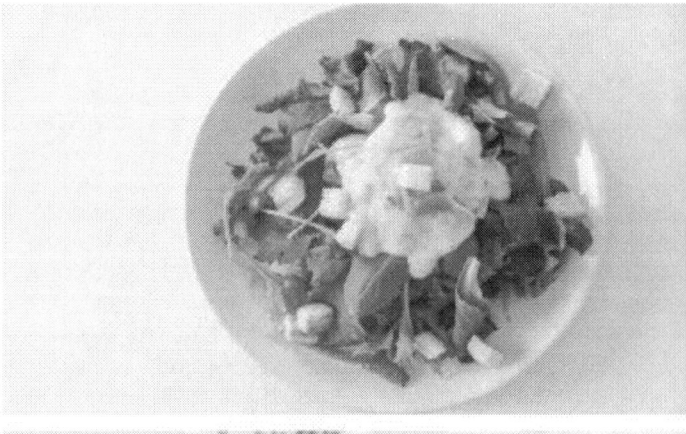
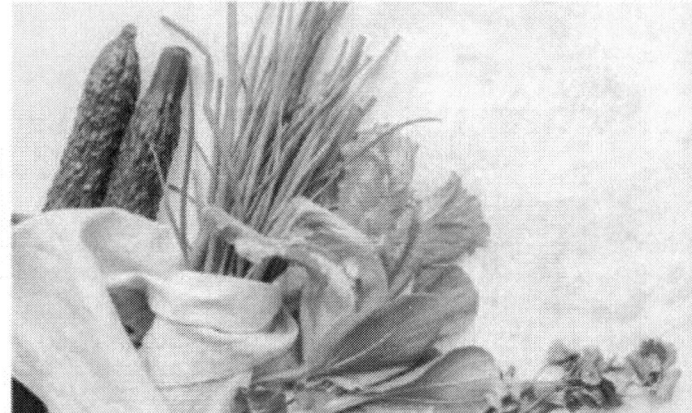

Benefits of the DASH Diet

The benefits of the DASH diet go beyond reducing hypertension and heart ailments.

CONTROLLING BLOOD PRESSURE: The force exerted on our blood vessels and organs when the blood passes through them is a measure of blood pressure in the human body. When the blood pressure increases beyond a certain level, it can lead to various bodily malfunctions, including heart failure.

Blood pressure is counted in two numbers: systolic pressure (pressure exerted in the blood vessels when the heart beats) and diastolic pressure (pressure exerted in the blood vessels when the heart is at rest). The normal blood systolic pressure in adults is below 120 mmHg, while the diastolic

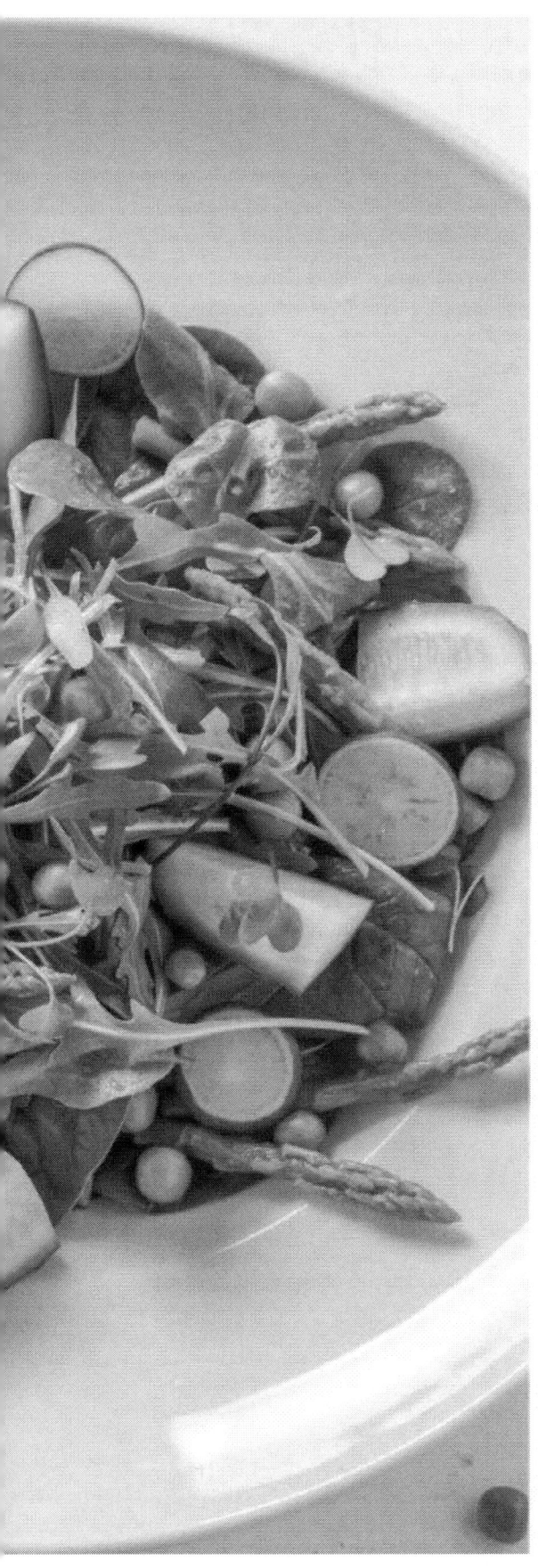

pressure is typically below 80 mmHg. Anyone over these limits is said to be suffering from high blood pressure.

The restriction of sodium intake and reliance on vegetables, healthy fat, lean meat, and fruits in the DASH diet greatly controls blood pressure. In fact, the lower one's salt intake, the lower one's blood pressure. Effective use of the DASH diet can c0ntrol the systolic blood pressure by an average change of 12 mmHg and can control the diastolic blood pressure by 5 mmHg.

The DASH diet is not reserved for people suffering from hypertension; it can also work well for people with normal blood pressure. The trick is to consume normal amounts of salt along with the dietary recommendations given in the DASH diet.

Weight loss: People with high blood pressure are advised to maintain their weight, as extra weight may translate into health complications. Obesity along with high blood pressure can lead to heart and organ failure.

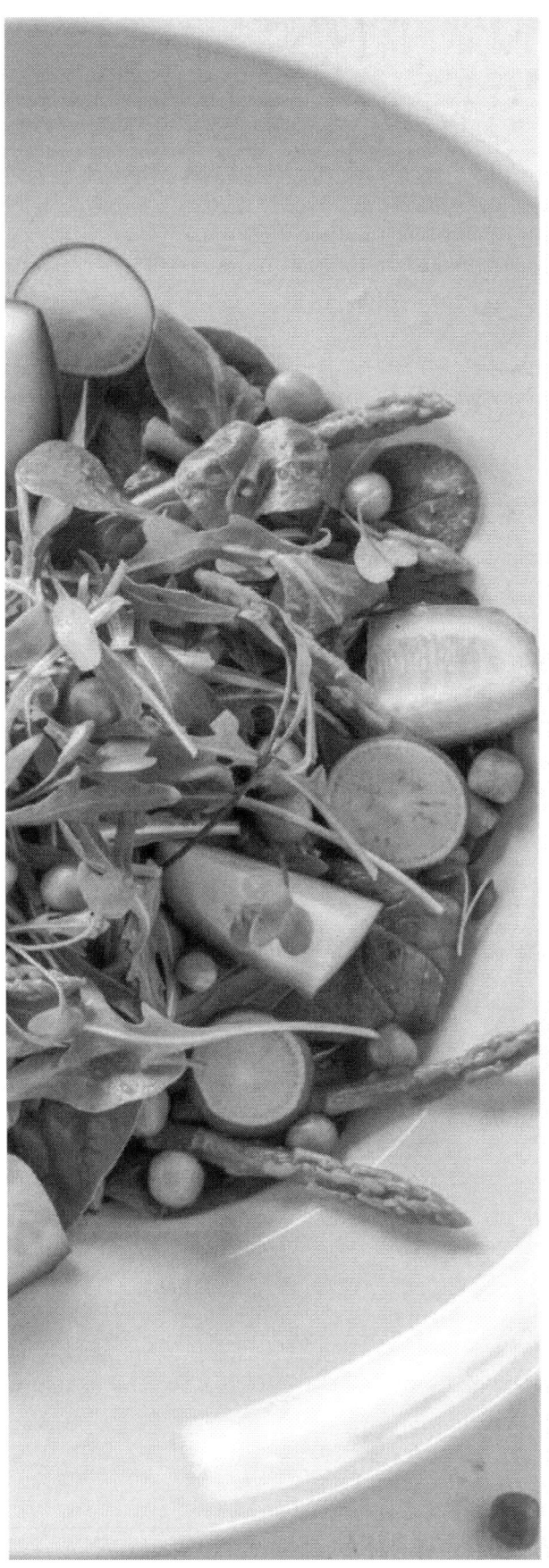

With the help of the DASH diet, one can lower their blood pressure while also lowering their weight. The credit for this goes to the healthy foods recommended in the DASH diet. The person is advised to cut down on their daily calorie count to lose weight.

Further, the DASH diet has shown signs of other health benefits:

FIGHTS CANCER RISK: People on the DASH diet have a lower risk of colorectal and breast cancers.

CHECKS METABOLIC SYNDROME: The diet reduces the risk of metabolic syndrome.

CONTROLS DIABETES: The diet is very beneficial for people with type 2 diabetes.

HEART DISEASES: The diet reduces the risk of heart disease and stroke.

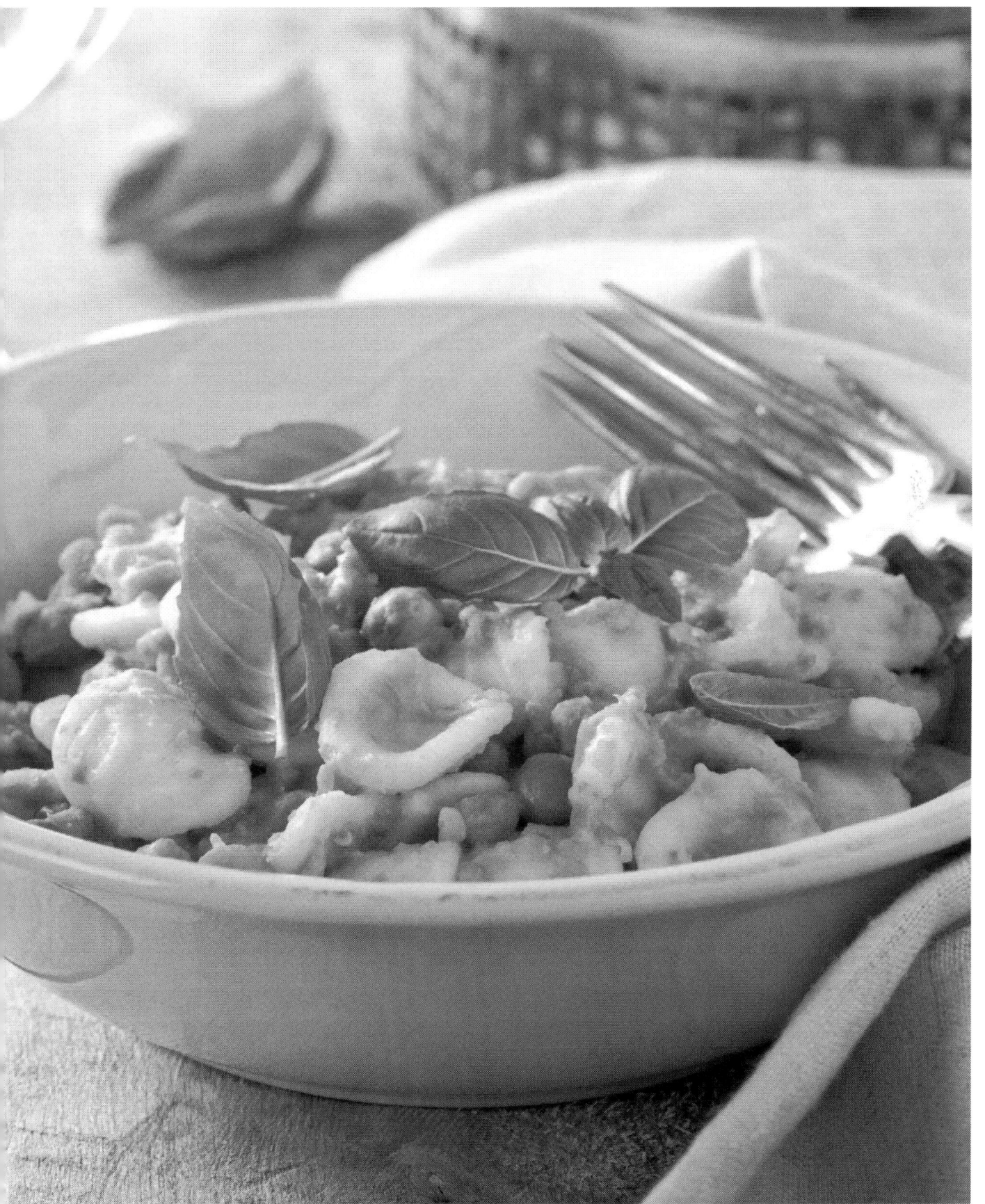

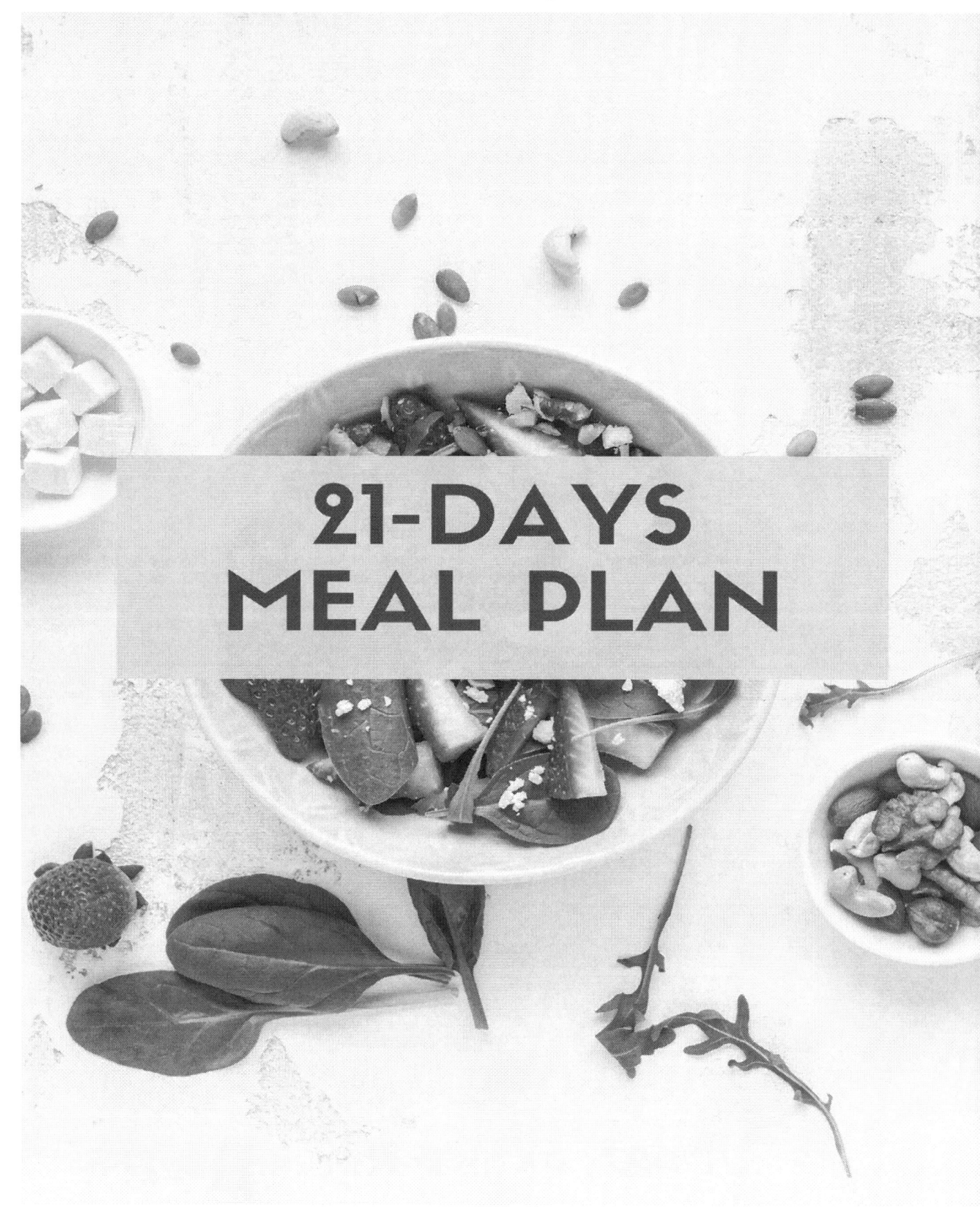

21-DAYS MEAL PLAN

Day 1
Breakfast – High-Calorie Breakfast Smoothie
Lunch – Asian-Style Pork Tenderloin
Dinner – Barley and Tomato Roast Risotto

Day 2
Breakfast – Overnight Refrigerated Oatmeal
Lunch – Baked Chicken with Herbed Wild Rice
Dinner – Easy Beef Brisket

Day 3
Breakfast – Cinnamon and Nutmeg French Toast
Lunch – Baked Cod Topped with Capers and Lemon
Dinner – Spiced Chipotle Shrimp

Day 4
Breakfast – Multi-Grain Hot Cereal
Lunch – Baked Red Sauce Macaroni
Dinner – Puttanesca Served with Brown Rice

Day 5
Breakfast – Cream Cheese and Strawberry Crepes
Lunch – Baked Salmon Topped with Asian Marinade
Dinner – Chicken Asparagus Penne

Day 6
Breakfast – Healthy Buckwheat Pancakes
Lunch – Classic Chicken Quesadillas
Dinner – Asian-Style Grilled Salmon

Day 7
Breakfast – Mushroom Spinach Frittata
Lunch – Pork Tenderloin Curry in Apple Cider
Dinner – Pork Medallions in Five Spices

Day 8
Breakfast – Sweet Potato Breakfast Waffles Topped with Blueberry Sauce
Lunch – Clams Fettuccine
Dinner – Baked Herb-Crusted Cod

Day 9
Breakfast – Healthy Baked Oatmeal
Lunch – Strip Steak with Mushroom Whiskey Sauce
Dinner – Roast Balsamic Chicken

Day 10
Breakfast – Blueberry Pancakes (Whole-Wheat)
Lunch – Creamy Polenta with Veggies
Dinner – Garlic and Broccoli Rigatoni

Day 11
Breakfast – Green Smoothie
Lunch – Chicken Salad with Balsamic Vinaigrette and Pineapple
Dinner – White Broiled Sea Bass

Day 12
Breakfast – Breakfast Muesli Bars
Lunch – Flank Steak and Roasted Corn Salad with Vinaigrette
Dinner – Easy Beef Stroganoff

Day 13
Breakfast – Fresh Mixed Fruit Smoothie
Lunch – Chicken Salad (Grilled) with Buttermilk Dressing
Dinner – Vegetarian Tofu Chili

Day 14
Breakfast – Banana and Oatmeal Pancakes
Lunch – Chicken Burritos
Dinner – Southwestern-Style Vegan Bowl

Day 15
Breakfast – Orange Vanilla Smoothie
Lunch – Brussels Sprouts with Lemon and Shallots
Dinner – Black-Eyed Creole-Style Peas

Day 16
Breakfast – Overnight Refrigerated Oatmeal
Lunch – Baked Chicken with Herbed Wild Rice
Dinner – Barley and Tomato Roast Risotto

Day 17
Breakfast – Mushroom Spinach Frittata
Lunch – Baked Salmon Topped with Asian Marinade
Dinner – Spiced Chipotle Shrimp

Day 18
Breakfast – Multi-Grain Hot Cereal
Lunch – Clams Fettuccine
Dinner – Chicken Asparagus Penne

Day 19
Breakfast – Blueberry Pancakes (Whole-Wheat)
Lunch – Chicken Salad with Balsamic Vinaigrette and Pineapple
Dinner – Pork Medallions in Five Spices

Day 20
Breakfast – Sweet Potato Breakfast Waffles Topped with Blueberry Sauce
Lunch – Chicken Burritos
Dinner Baked Herb-Crusted Cod

Day 21
Breakfast – Green Smoothie
Lunch – Brussels Sprouts with Lemon and Shallots
Dinner – Vegetarian Tofu Chili

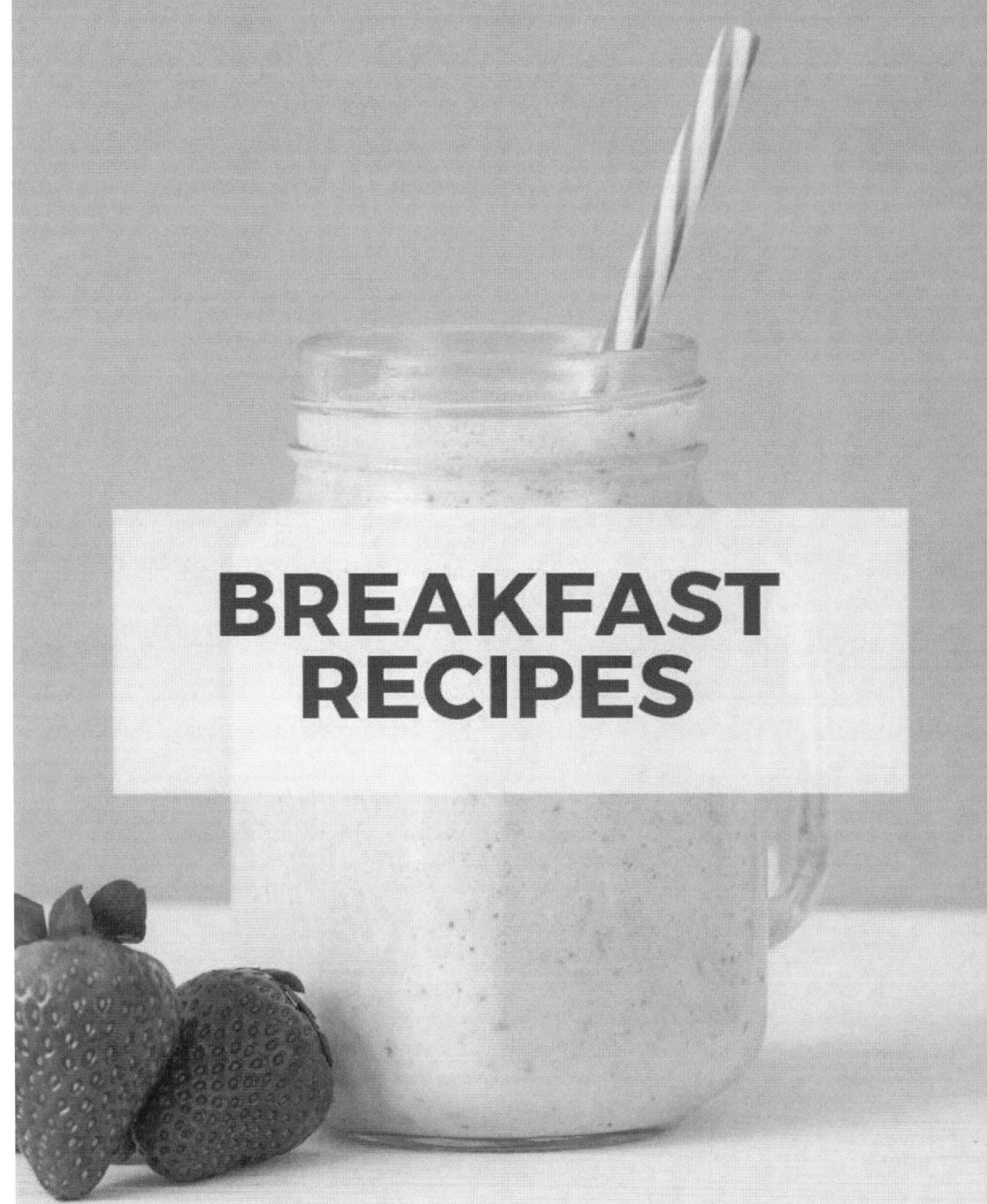

BREAKFAST RECIPES

BANANA AND OATMEAL PANCAKES

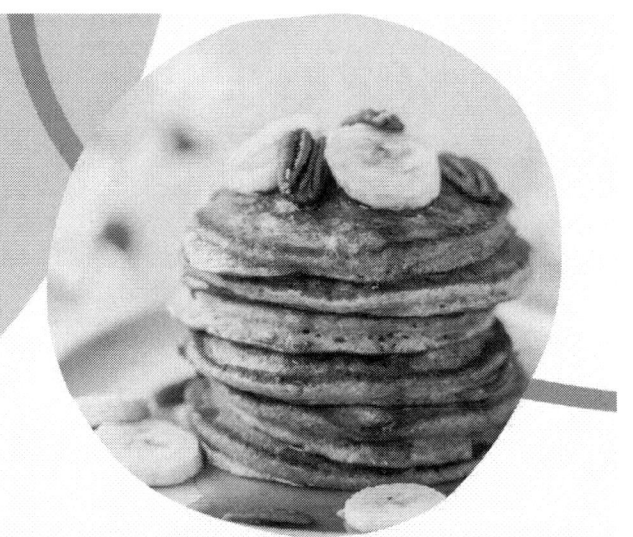

GENERAL INFO

Serving size: 3
Servings per recipe: 4
Calories: 288 calories per serving
Total time: 1 hour 5 minutes

INGREDIENTS

Rolled oats (old-fashioned) – ½ cup
Hot water – 1 cup
Canola oil – 2 tablespoons
Brown sugar – 2 tablespoons
Whole-wheat flour – ½ cup
All-purpose flour – ½ cup
Baking powder – 1 ½ teaspoons
Baking soda – ¼ teaspoon
Salt – ¼ teaspoon
Ground cinnamon – ¼ teaspoon
Skim milk – ½ cup
Plain yogurt (fat-free) – ¼ cup
Banana (mashed) – 1
Egg – 1

NUTRITION INFO

Protein – 9 g
Sodium – 453 mg
Carbohydrates – 45 g
Fat – 9 g

BANANA AND OATMEAL PANCAKES

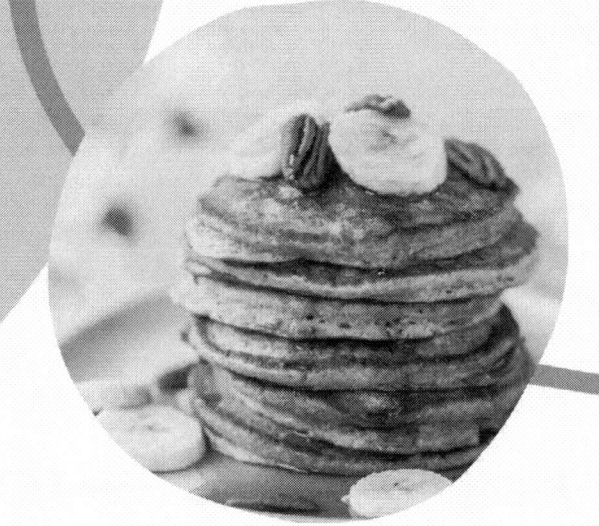

DIRECTIONS

1. Start by taking a large glass bowl and adding in the hot water and rolled oats. Set aside for a couple of minutes. Give it a mix.
2. Add in the sugar and oil and mix until well combined. Set aside until it cools down a bit.
3. Take a medium-sized bowl and add in the wheat flour, all-purpose flour, baking soda, baking powder, ground cinnamon, and salt. Use a whisk to mix all the ingredients well.
4. Also, add the yogurt, banana, and milk to the oats mixture and mix until all ingredients are well incorporated.
5. Combine the oat mixture and flour mixture. Also, beat in an egg and mix well.
6. Take a nonstick griddle and place it on a medium-high flame. Grease it with nonstick cooking spray and let it heat through.
7. Once the griddle is hot enough, use a ¼ measuring cup to scoop out the batter and drop it on the griddle. Cook for around 2 minutes; flip over and cook for another 3 minutes. Repeat the process with the remaining pancake batter.
8. Serve hot!

An Appeal from the Publisher

Hello wonderful reader!

We hope you are enjoying this book.

We wanted to let you know that you have made an impact on many lives by reading this book.

Just to give you a brief introduction: We are a small publishing company with a team of 8 writers and 2 editors.

Most of our employees come from financially weaker section and our company is the only means they support their families. This is our way of giving back to the society.

We don't have the giant advertising budgets that many other publishers and businesses do online.

So, one way that you can really support our mission and our business is by leaving us a review on this book.

For a small company like us, getting reviews (especially on Amazon) means we can submit our books for advertising.

This means we can actually sell a few copies from time to time and make a bigger impact on the society as a whole. So, every review means a lot to us.

We can't THANK YOU enough for this!

BLUEBERRY PANCAKES (WHOLE-WHEAT)

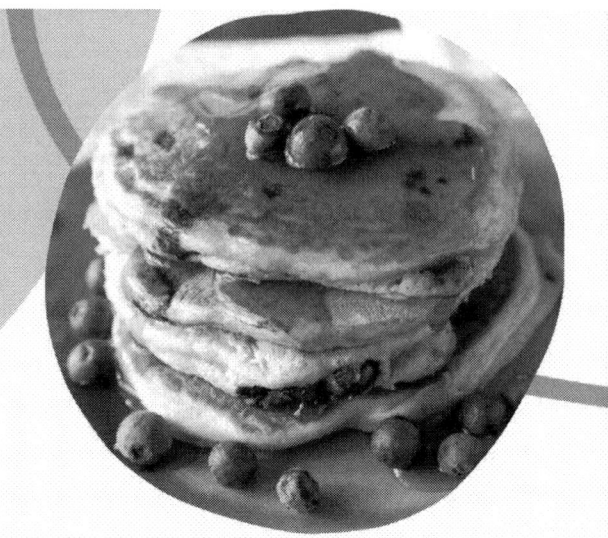

GENERAL INFO

Serving size: 2
Servings per recipe: 6
Calories: 158 calories per serving

INGREDIENTS

Whole-wheat flour (white) – 1 1/3 cups
Baking powder – 2 teaspoons
Sugar – 1 tablespoon
Cinnamon – ½ teaspoon
Skim milk – 1 1/3 cups
Egg (lightly beaten) – 1
Canola oil – 1 tablespoon
Fresh blueberries – 1 cup

NUTRITION INFO

Protein – 6 g
Sodium – 240 mg
Carbohydrates – 28 g
Fat – 4 g

BLUEBERRY PANCAKES (WHOLE-WHEAT)

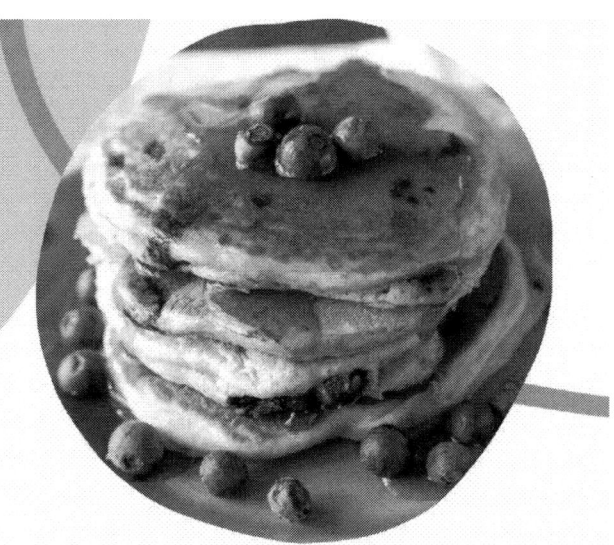

DIRECTIONS

1. Take a large glass bowl and add in the whole-wheat flour, sugar, cinnamon, and baking powder. Mix until well combined.
2. Take another bowl and add in the milk, oil, and eggs. Whisk well until all ingredients are nicely incorporated.
3. Transfer the egg mixture to the flour mixture and mix well.
4. Now toss in the blueberries and gently fold them into the mixture.
5. Take a nonstick griddle and place it on a medium-high flame. Grease the griddle with nonstick cooking spray and let it heat through.
6. Once the griddle is hot enough, take a measuring cup and scoop out ¼ cup of prepared batter. Empty it onto the griddle. Cook for about 2 minutes on each side. Repeat the process with the remaining batter.
7. Serve right away!

BREAKFAST MUESLI BARS

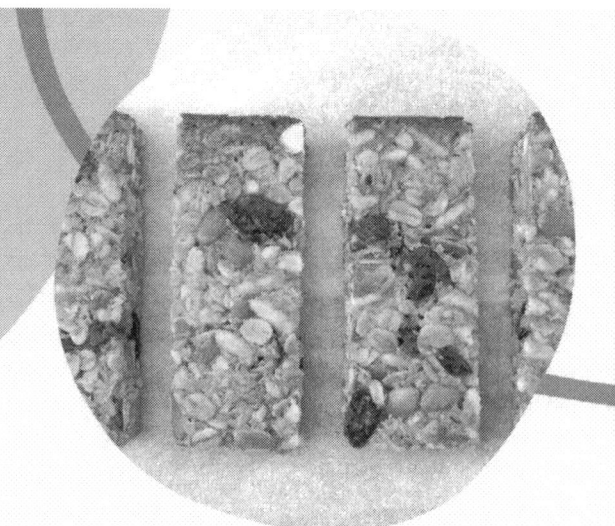

GENERAL INFO

Serving size: 1
Servings per recipe: 24
Calories: 169 calories per serving
Total time: 40 minutes

INGREDIENTS

Rolled oats (old-fashioned) – 2 ½ cups
Soy flour – ½ cup
Dry milk (fat-free) – ½ cup
Wheat germ (toasted) – ½ cup
Toasted almonds (sliced) – ½ cup
Dried apples (chopped) – ½ cup
Raisins – ½ cup
Salt – ½ teaspoon
Dark honey – 1 cup
Natural peanut butter (unsalted) – ½ cup
Olive oil – 1 tablespoon
Vanilla extract – 2 teaspoons

NUTRITION INFO

Protein – 5 g
Sodium – 81 mg
Carbohydrates – 26 g
Fat – 5 g

BREAKFAST MUESLI BARS

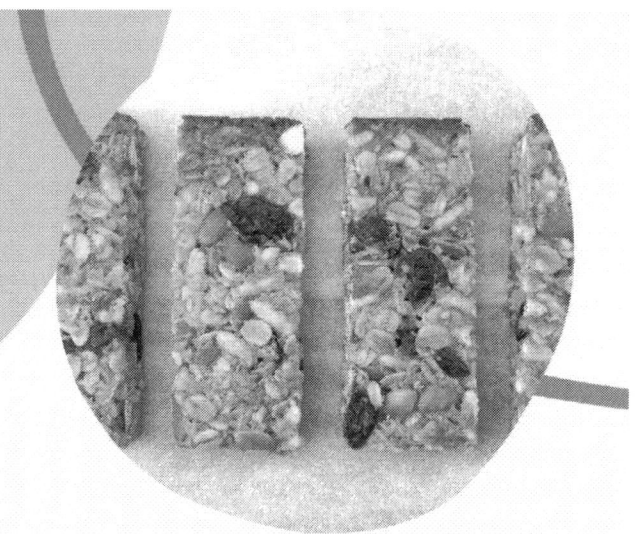

DIRECTIONS

1. Begin by preheating the oven by setting the temperature to 325 degrees Fahrenheit.
2. Take a 9x13 baking dish and grease it with nonstick cooking spray. Set it aside
3. In a large glass bowl, add in the flour, oats, dry milk, almonds, wheat germ, apples, salt, and raisins. Mix well and set aside.
4. Take a small saucepan and place it on a medium-low flame. Pour in the olive oil and let it get warm.
5. Add in the peanut butter and honey and mix until it is well combined; let it come to a boil.
6. Once the mixture boils, stir in the vanilla. Remove from the flame.
7. Pour the prepared honey mixture into the flour and oats mixture. Mix quickly until the ingredients are perfectly combined. Make sure there are no lumps at all.
8. Transfer the mixture to the greased baking dish and press to get rid of any air pockets.
9. Place the baking dish into the preheated oven and bake for around 25 minutes.
10. Once done, remove the dish from the oven and place it on a wire rack. Let it rest for around 10 minutes.
11. Use a sharp knife to cut 24 equal-sized bars. Remove them carefully once cut. Place the bars on the wire rack until they are completely cooled.
12. The bars can be stored in the fridge in an airtight glass container.

CINNAMON AND NUTMEG FRENCH TOAST

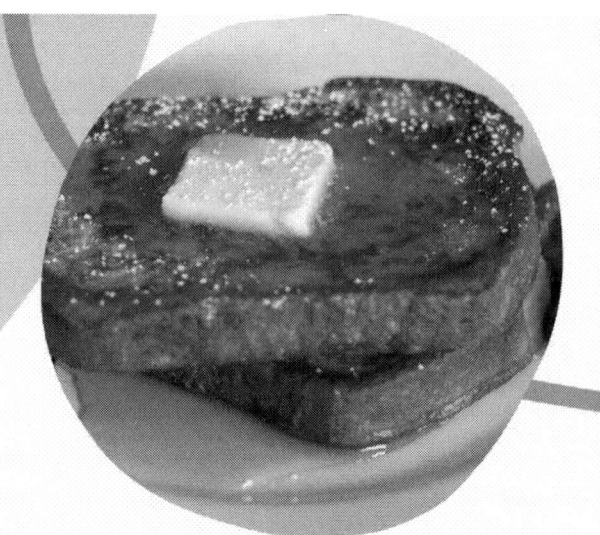

GENERAL INFO

Serving size: 2
Servings per recipe: 2
Calories: 299 calories per serving
Total time: 40 minutes

INGREDIENTS

Egg whites – 4
Vanilla – 1 teaspoon
Nutmeg (ground) – ⅛ teaspoon
Cinnamon bread – 4 slices
Cinnamon (ground) – ¼ teaspoon
Maple syrup – ¼ cup

NUTRITION INFO

Protein – 11 g
Sodium – 334 mg
Carbohydrates – 57 g
Fat – 3 g

CINNAMON AND NUTMEG FRENCH TOAST

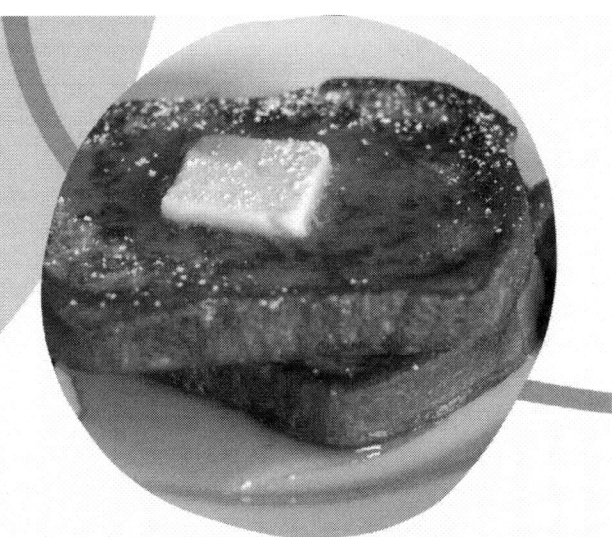

DIRECTIONS

1. Start by taking a small bowl and adding in the egg whites, nutmeg, and vanilla. Whisk well until all ingredients are nicely combined and smooth in texture.
2. Take a nonstick griddle and place it on a medium flame. Grease it with cooking spray.
3. Take the bread slice and dip it into the prepared egg mixture. Make sure both sides are nicely coated.
4. Once the griddle is hot enough, place the bread slice dipped into the egg onto the griddle. Sprinkle cinnamon on top and cook for 5 minutes. Flip over and cook for another 5 minutes. Repeat the process with the remaining 2 slices.
5. Once done, transfer the French toast onto the plate.
6. Finish by sprinkling a teaspoon of powdered sugar and a drizzle with 2 tablespoons of maple syrup.
7. Serve right away!

CREAM CHEESE AND STRAWBERRY CREPES

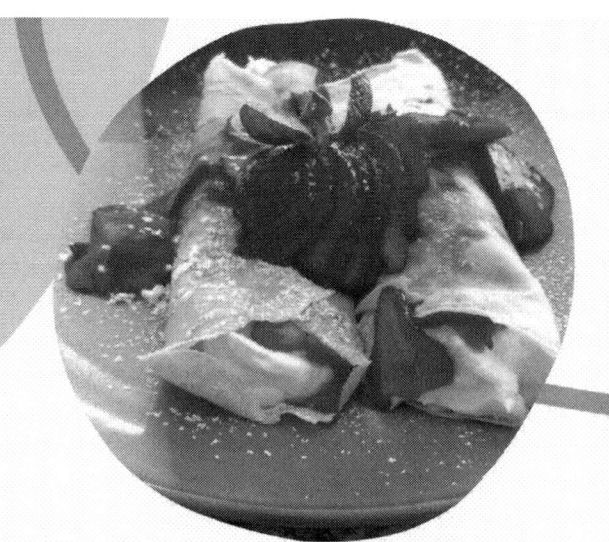

GENERAL INFO

Serving size: ½
Servings per recipe: 4
Calories: 143 calories per serving
Total time: minutes

INGREDIENTS

Cream cheese (softened) – 4 tablespoons
Powdered sugar (sifted) – 2 tablespoons
Vanilla extract – 2 teaspoons
Prepackaged crepes (8-inch diameter) – 2
Strawberries (sliced) – 8

For garnish:
Powdered sugar – 1 teaspoon
Caramel sauce (warmed) – 2 tablespoons

NUTRITION INFO

Protein – 3 g
Sodium – 161 mg
Carbohydrates – 17 g
Fat – 7 g

CREAM CHEESE AND STRAWBERRY CREPES

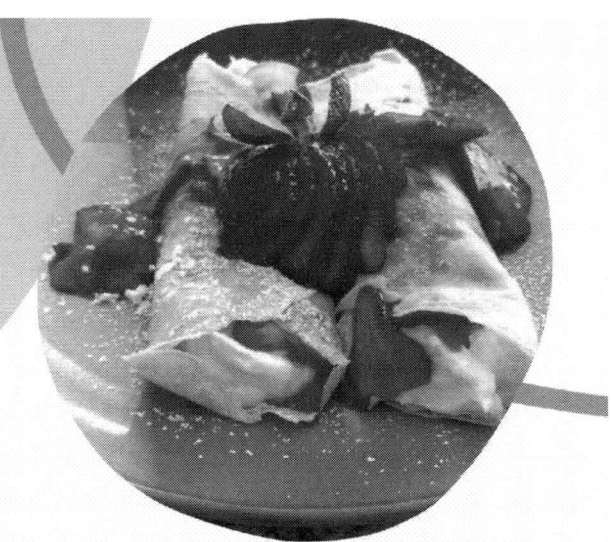

DIRECTIONS

1. Begin by preheating the oven by setting the temperature to 325 degrees Fahrenheit.
2. Take a baking dish and gently grease it with nonstick cooking spray. Set aside.
3. Take a large glass mixing bowl and add in the cream cheese. Use an electric hand mixer to blend until the cheese is smooth.
4. Add in the vanilla and powdered sugar and continue to mix until all ingredients are nicely incorporated.
5. Place the crepes on a flat surface and top each with half of the cream cheese mixture. Spread it evenly and further place the sliced strawberries on each of the crepes.
6. Take one end of the crepe and fold it into a roll. Roll the second crepe the same way and place it into the greased baking dish.
7. Place the dish into the preheated oven and bake for 10 minutes. The crepes should be lightly browned.
8. Once done, take out the baking dish and use a turner or tong to remove the crepes. Place the crepes onto a wooden chopping block and cut them in half.
9. Transfer the crepes onto a serving platter and garnish with a sprinkle of powdered sugar. Finish with a drizzle of the caramel sauce.
10. Serve!

FRESH MIXED FRUIT SMOOTHIE

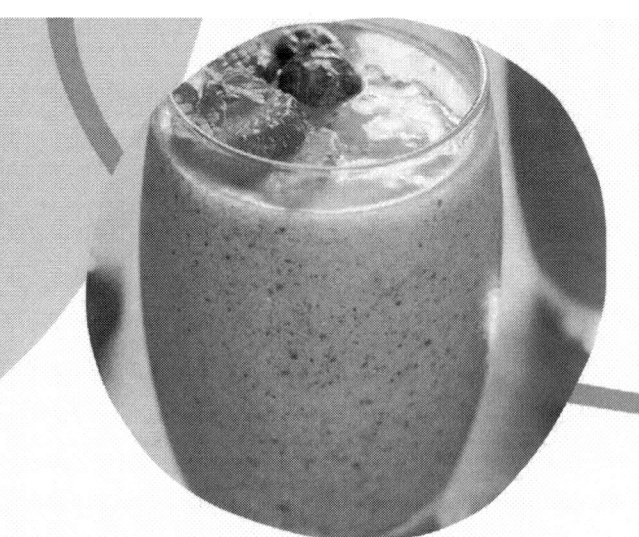

GENERAL INFO

Serving size: 8 ounces
Servings per recipe: 4
Calories: 72 calories per serving
Total time: 5 minutes

INGREDIENTS

Pineapple chunks (fresh) – 1 cup
Cantaloupe chunks – ½ cup
Strawberries (fresh) – 1 cup
Orange juice – 2 oranges
Cold water – 1 cup
Honey – 1 tablespoon

NUTRITION INFO

Protein – 1 g
Sodium – 7 mg
Carbohydrates – 17 g
Fat – 0 g

DIRECTIONS

1. Start by adding the pineapple chunks, cantaloupe chunks, strawberries, orange juice, honey, and cold water to the blender.
2. Blend the ingredients into a smooth puree-like consistency.
3. Transfer the smoothie into the glasses and serve!

GREEN SMOOTHIE

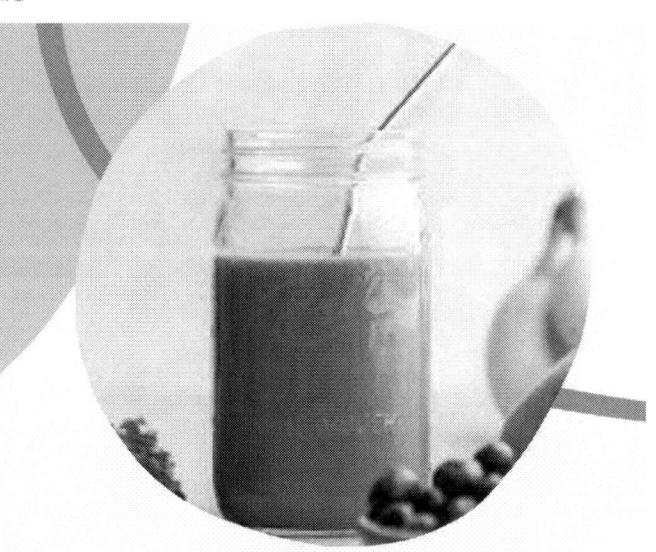

GENERAL INFO

Serving size: 6 ounces
Servings per recipe: 4
Calories: 64 calories per serving
Total time: 5 minutes

NUTRITION INFO

Protein – 1 g
Sodium – 5 mg
Carbohydrates – 12 g
Fat – 0 g

INGREDIENTS

Banana – 1
Lemon juice – 4 tablespoons
Strawberries – ½ cup
Blueberries or blackberries – ½ cup
Baby spinach (fresh) – 2 ounces
Fresh mint – to taste
Cold water – 1 cup

DIRECTIONS

1. Take a blender and add in the banana, lemon juice, strawberries, blueberries or blackberries, baby spinach, fresh mint, and cold water.
2. Blend into a smooth puree-like consistency.
3. Transfer into a tall glass and serve cold!

HEALTHY BAKED OATMEAL

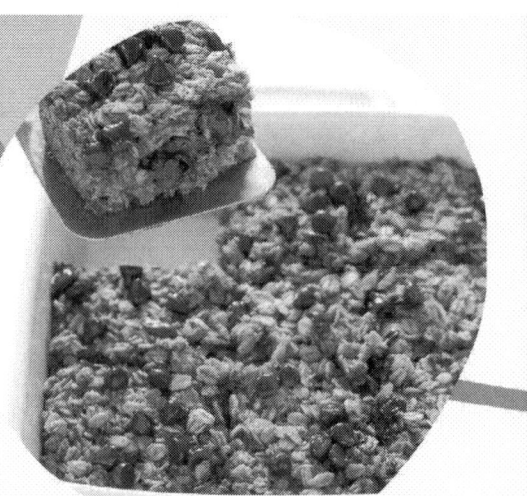

GENERAL INFO

Serving size: ¾ cup
Servings per recipe: 8
Calories: 196 calories per serving
Total time: 35 minutes

INGREDIENTS

Canola oil – 1 tablespoon
Applesauce (unsweetened) – ½ cup
Brown sugar – 1/3 cup
Egg whites – 4
Rolled oats (uncooked) – 3 cups
Baking powder – 2 teaspoons
Cinnamon – 1 teaspoon
Skim milk – 1 cup

NUTRITION INFO

Protein – 7 g
Sodium – 105 mg
Carbohydrates – 33 g
Fat – 4 g

HEALTHY BAKED OATMEAL

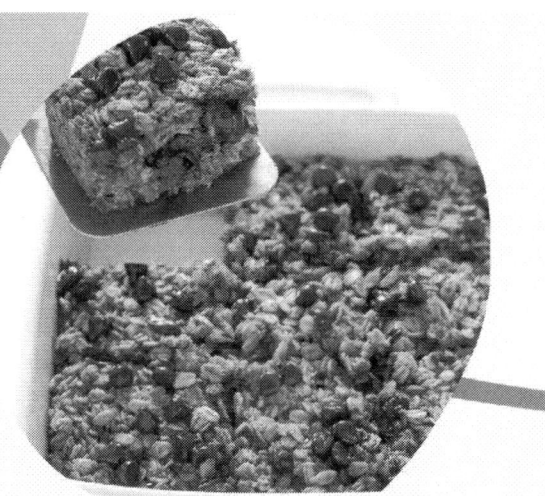

DIRECTIONS

1. Start by taking a large glass bowl and adding in the oil, sugar, egg whites, and applesauce. Mix well using a whisk.
2. Now add in the rolled oats, cinnamon, and baking powder. Whisk until well combined.
3. Take a baking dish measuring 9x13 and generously grease with butter or cooking spray.
4. Transfer the prepared mixture into the baking dish and place in the oven.
5. Bake for 30 minutes at 350 degrees Fahrenheit.
6. Once done, take the oatmeal out of the oven and serve!

HEALTHY BUCKWHEAT PANCAKES

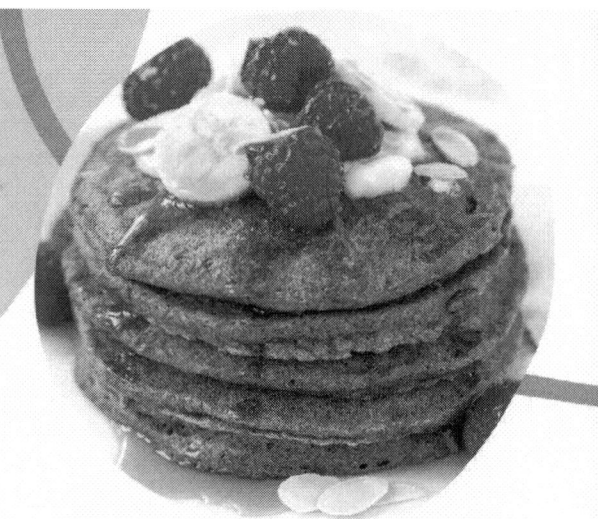

GENERAL INFO

Serving size: 2
Servings per recipe: 6
Calories: 143 calories per serving
Total time: 30 minutes

INGREDIENTS

Egg whites – 2
Canola oil – 1 tablespoon
Milk (fat-free) – ½ cup
All-purpose flour – ½ cup
Buckwheat flour – ½ cup
Baking powder – 1 tablespoon
Sugar – 1 tablespoon
Sparkling water – ½ cup
Fresh strawberries (sliced) – 3 cups

NUTRITION INFO

Protein – 5 g
Sodium – 150 mg
Carbohydrates – 24 g
Fat – 3 g

HEALTHY BUCKWHEAT PANCAKES

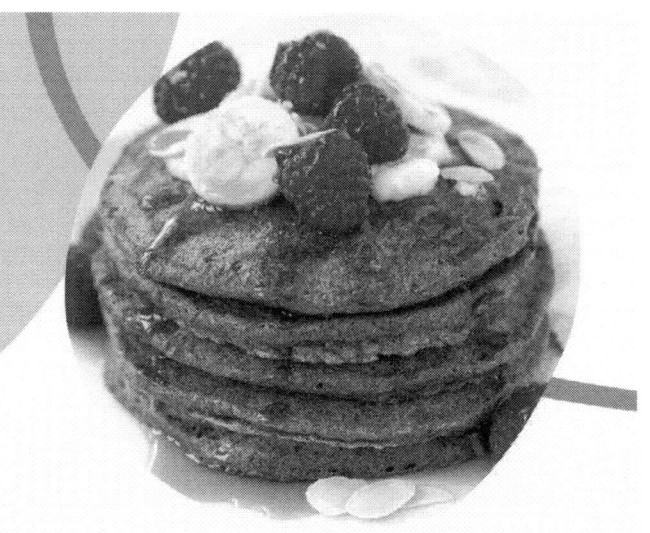

DIRECTIONS

1. Take a small glass mixing bowl and add in the egg whites, milk, and canola oil. Whisk until all ingredients are well combined.
2. Take another glass mixing bowl and add in the all-purpose flour, buckwheat flour, sugar, and baking powder. Use a whisk to mix all the ingredients well.
3. Add in the egg whites and sparkling water and whisk into a smooth batter-like consistency. Set aside.
4. Take a nonstick griddle and place it over a medium flame. Grease it with nonstick cooking spray and let it heat through.
5. Use a measuring cup to scoop ½ cup of batter and drop it on the griddle. Cook for about 2 minutes. Flip over and cook for another 2 minutes. Repeat the process with the rest of the batter.
6. Transfer onto a serving platter and top with sliced strawberries.
7. Serve right away!

HIGH-CALORIE BREAKFAST SMOOTHIE

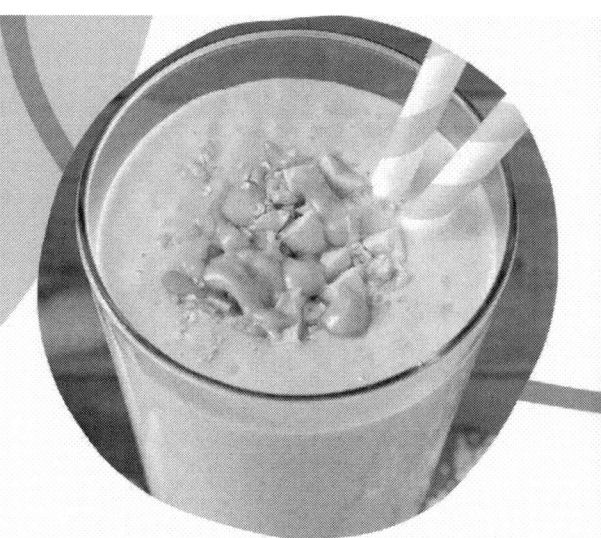

GENERAL INFO

Serving size: 1
Servings per recipe: 1
Calories: 608 calories per serving
Total time: 5 minutes

INGREDIENTS

Vanilla yogurt – 1 cup
2 percent milk – 1 cup
Banana – 1 medium
Wheat germ – 2 tablespoons
Protein powder – 2 tablespoons

NUTRITION INFO

Protein – 32 g
Sodium – 301 mg
Carbohydrates – 75 g
Fat – 20 g

DIRECTIONS

1. Begin by peeling the banana and cutting it into small chunks.
2. Take a blender and add in the chopped banana chunks, yogurt, milk, protein powder, and wheat germ. Blend until it becomes smooth.
3. Transfer into a tall glass and top with fresh mint leaves for extra freshness.

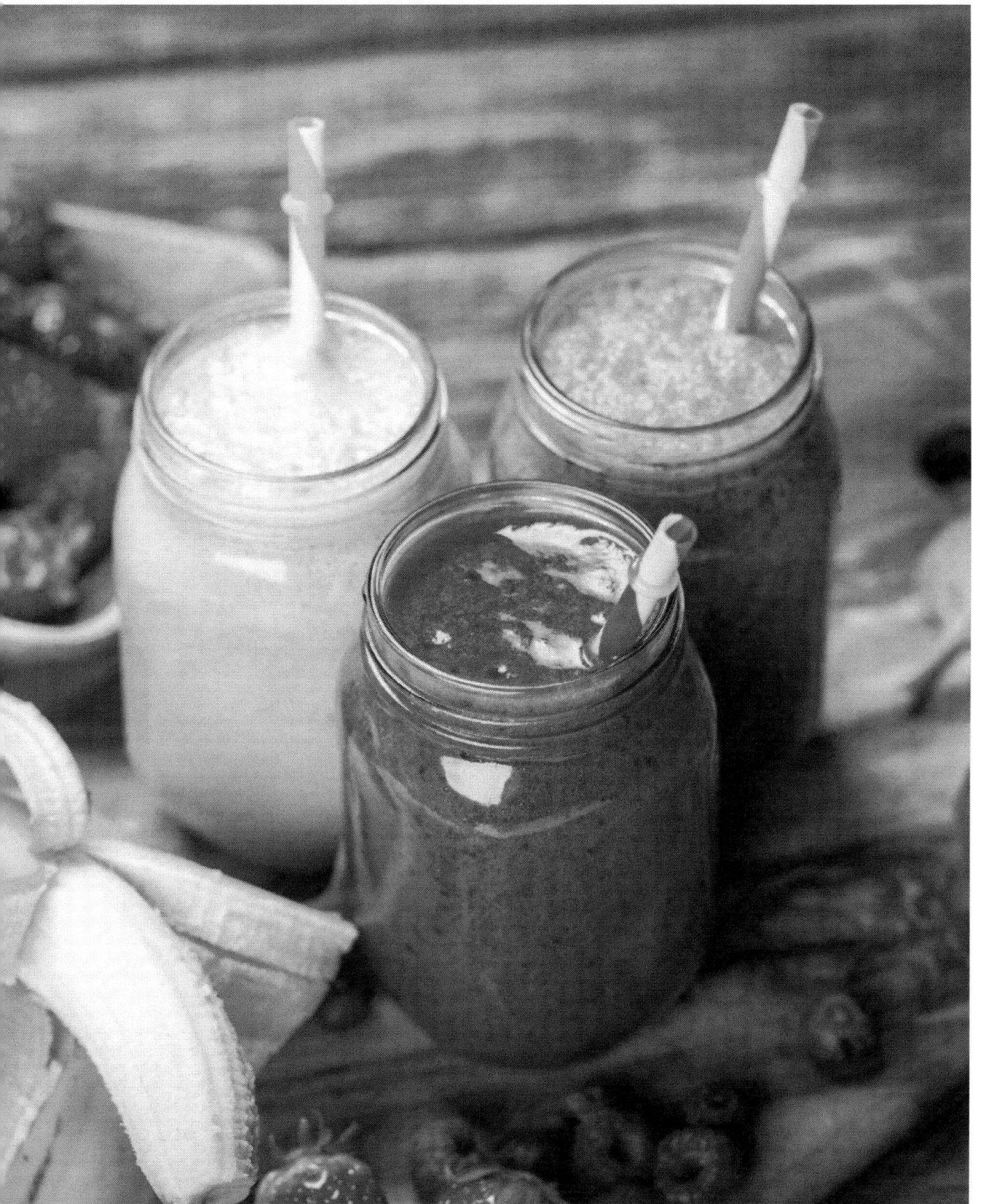

MULTI-GRAIN HOT CEREAL

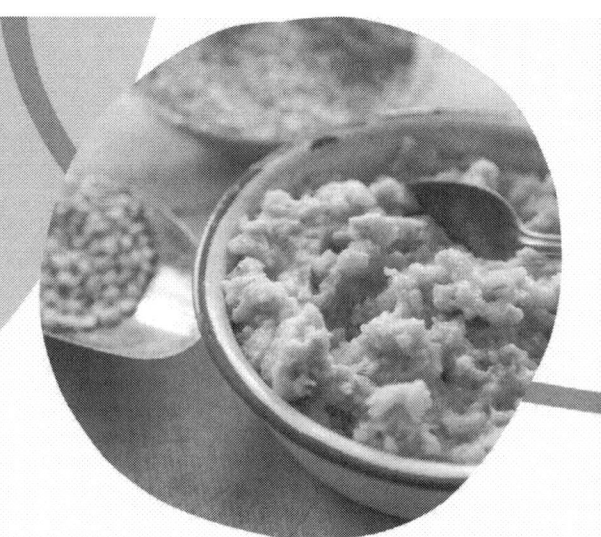

GENERAL INFO

Serving size: ½ cup
Servings per recipe: 14
Calories: 114 calories per serving
Total time: 50 minutes

INGREDIENTS

Pearl barley (uncooked) – ½ cup
Red wheat berries (uncooked) – ½ cup
Brown rice (uncooked) – ½ cup
Steel-cut oats (uncooked) – ¼ cup
Quinoa (uncooked) – 3 tablespoons
Flaxseed – 2 tablespoons
Kosher salt – ½ teaspoon
Water – 1 ½ quart
Parsley (finely chopped) – for garnishing

NUTRITION INFO

Protein – 4 g
Sodium – 74 mg
Carbohydrates – 21 g
Fat – 1 g

MULTI-GRAIN HOT CEREAL

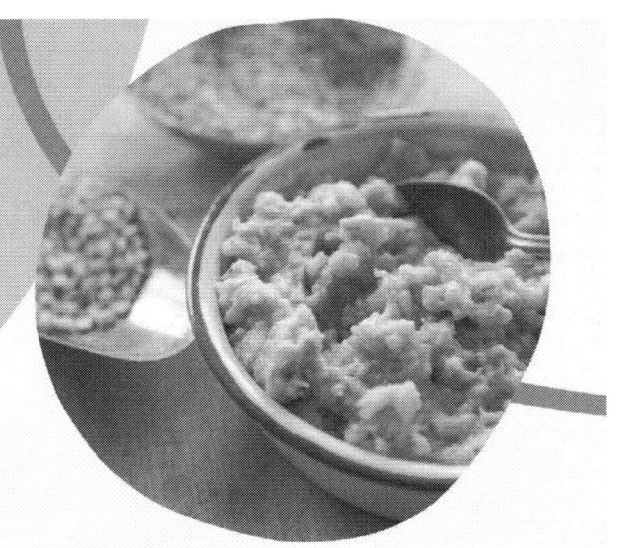

DIRECTIONS

1. Take a large nonstick saucepan and place it over a medium flame.
2. Add in the barley, rice, wheat berries, oats, flaxseed, salt, and quinoa. Mix well.
3. Pour the water into the sauce and give it a nice mix. Keep stirring until the cereal comes to a boil.
4. Once the cereal begins to boil, reduce the flame to low and cook for about 45 minutes. Keep stirring to prevent it from sticking to the bottom.
5. Turn off the flame and transfer to a serving bowl.
6. Garnish with fresh parsley or cilantro.

MUSHROOM SPINACH FRITTATA

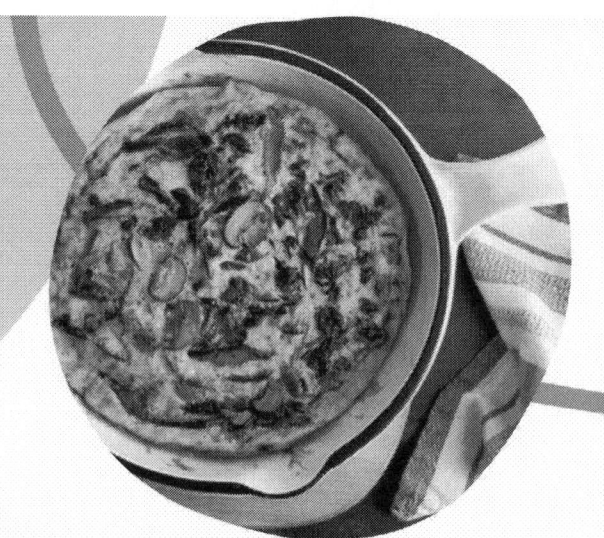

GENERAL INFO

Serving size: 1
Servings per recipe: 6
Calories: 106 calories per serving
Total time: 40 minutes

INGREDIENTS

Garlic (minced) – 3 cloves
Onion (chopped) – 1 cup
Olive oil – 1 teaspoon
Mushrooms (sliced) – ½ pound
Dried thyme – ½ teaspoon
Fresh spinach – 10 ounces
Water – 1 tablespoon
Egg substitute – 10 eggs equivalent
Dried dill – 1 teaspoon
Black pepper – ¼ teaspoon
Feta cheese – ¼ cup

NUTRITION INFO

Protein – 14 g
Sodium – 290 mg
Carbohydrates – 8 g
Fat – 2 g

MUSHROOM SPINACH FRITTATA

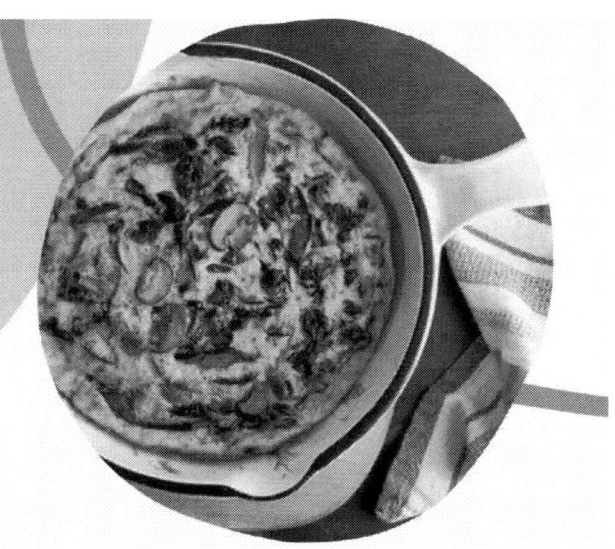

DIRECTIONS

1. Begin by preheating the oven by setting the temperature to 350 degrees Fahrenheit.
2. Take a cast-iron skillet and place it over a medium flame. Pour in the olive oil and heat until it becomes warm.
3. Add in the onion and garlic and sauté for around 5 minutes. Toss in the mushrooms and sauté for 5 more minutes.
4. Once done, remove from the flame and set it aside.
5. Take another large skillet and place the spinach into the same. Also, add a tablespoon of water. Use a lid to cover the skillet and cook for a couple of minutes. Once done, transfer the spinach into a colander. Use your hands to squeeze out any excess water. Add to the mushroom mixture and mix well.
6. Take a large glass mixing bowl and add in the egg substitute, pepper, and dill. Mix well. Also, add in the feta cheese and mushroom-spinach mixture. Mix until well combined.
7. Use a tissue to wipe any excess oil from the cast iron skillet. Generously coat the skillet with nonstick cooking spray.

MUSHROOM SPINACH FRITTATA

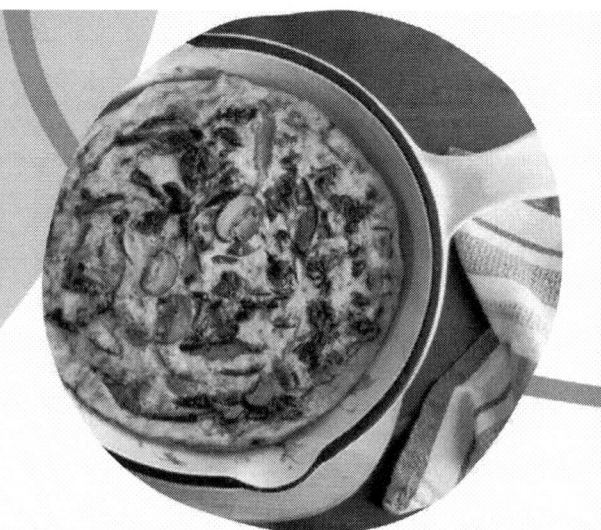

DIRECTIONS

8. Place the greased skillet on a medium flame and let it heat through. Pour in the egg mixture and place it into the preheated oven.
9. Cook the frittata for 20 minutes, checking every 5 minutes. Use a toothpick to check if the egg is firm enough.
10. Once baked, take out the frittata from the oven and flip it over onto a wooden black.
11. Cut into 6 equal picccs and serve right away.

ORANGE VANILLA SMOOTHIE

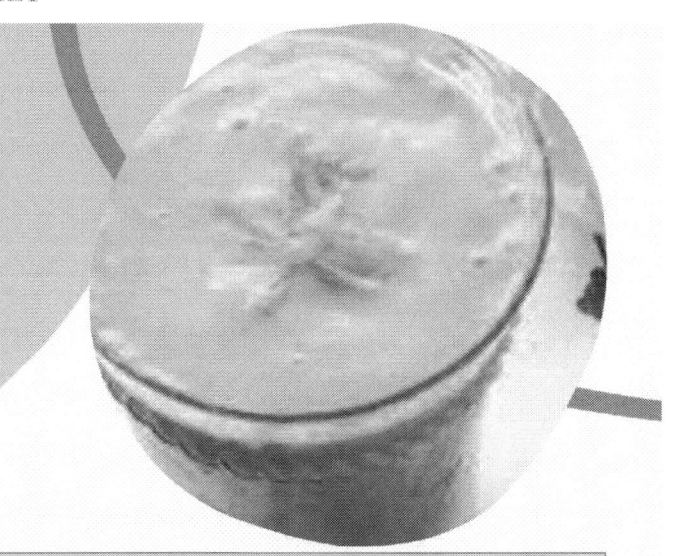

GENERAL INFO

Serving size: 1 cup
Servings per recipe: 4
Calories: 101 calories per serving
Total time: 5 minutes

NUTRITION INFO

Protein – 3 g
Sodium – 40 mg
Carbohydrates – 20 g
Fat – 1 g

INGREDIENTS

Orange juice – 1 ½ cups
Light soy milk (vanilla) – 1 cup
Soft tofu – 1/3 cup
Dark honey – 1 tablespoon
Orange zest (grated) – 1 teaspoon
Vanilla extract – ½ teaspoon
Ice cubes – 5
Orange segments (peeled) – 4

DIRECTIONS

1. Begin by taking a blender and combining the orange juice, tofu, soy milk, orange zest, honey, ice cubes, and vanilla.
2. Blend the ingredients for 30 seconds until you have a puree-like consistency. The puree should be smooth.
3. Pour the smoothie into a tall glass and top it with pieces of orange segments.
4. Serve chilled!

OVERNIGHT REFRIGERATED OATMEAL

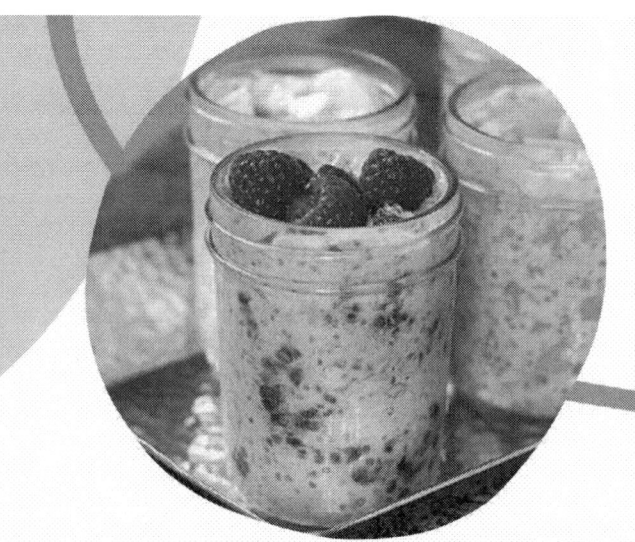

GENERAL INFO

Serving size: 1
Servings per recipe: 1
Calories: 193 calories per serving
Total time: 8 hours

INGREDIENTS

Soy milk – 1/3 cup
Applesauce (unsweetened) – ¼ cup
Rolled oats (old-fashioned) – ¼ cup
Greek plain yogurt (low-fat) – ¼ cup
Apples (diced) – ¼ cup
Chia seeds (dried) – 1 ½ teaspoons
Cinnamon – ¼ teaspoon

NUTRITION INFO

Protein – 11 g
Sodium – 89 mg
Carbohydrates – 30 g
Fat – 4 g

OVERNIGHT REFRIGERATED OATMEAL

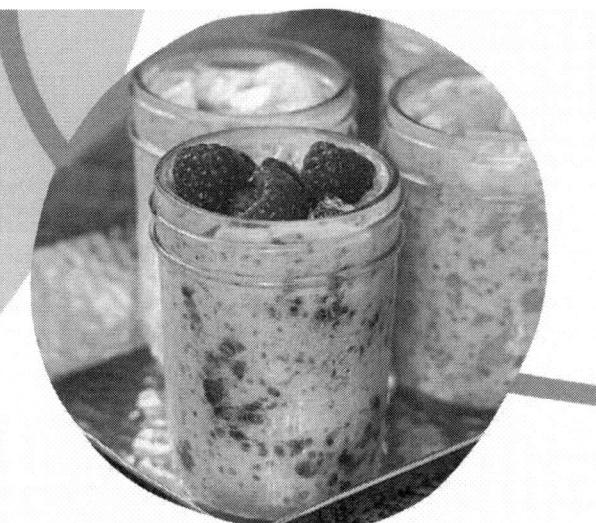

DIRECTIONS

1. Take a 500 ml Mason jar and add in the soy milk [almond milk], unsweetened applesauce, rolled oats, low-fat Greek yogurt, diced apples, dried chia seeds, and cinnamon.
2. Close the lid and shake well until all ingredients are nicely combined.
3. Place the Mason jar into the refrigerator for at least 8 hours or overnight.
4. Serve with fresh fruit toppings of your choice or enjoy as-is.

Emma's version
- old fashioned oats
- plain yogurt
- milk
- vanilla
- maple syrup *
- apple
- cinnamon
- salt

SWEET POTATO BREAKFAST WAFFLES

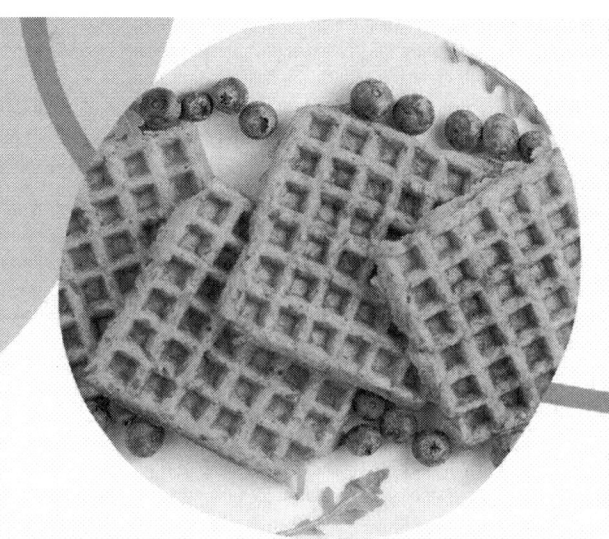

GENERAL INFO

Serving size: 1
Servings per recipe: 6
Calories: 222 calories per serving
Total time: 50 minutes

NUTRITION INFO

Protein – 5 g
Sodium – 192 mg
Carbohydrates – 37 g
Fat – 6 g

INGREDIENTS

For waffles:
Sweet potato (peeled and diced) – 1/3 cup
All-purpose flour – ¾ cup
Whole-wheat flour – ¼ cup
Cornmeal – ¼ cup
Baking powder – 1 tablespoon
Salt – ½ teaspoon
Ground cinnamon – ⅛ teaspoon
Ground ginger – ⅛ teaspoon
Plain soy milk – 1 cup
Light molasses – 2 tablespoons
Olive oil – 2 tablespoons
Egg white – 1

For blueberry sauce:
Fresh blueberries – 1 ½ cups
Water – 2 tablespoons
Lemon juice (freshly squeezed) – 1 tablespoon
Grated lemon zest – 1 teaspoon
Honey – 1 tablespoon
Light molasses – 1 tablespoon
Ground cloves – a pinch

SWEET POTATO BREAKFAST WAFFLES

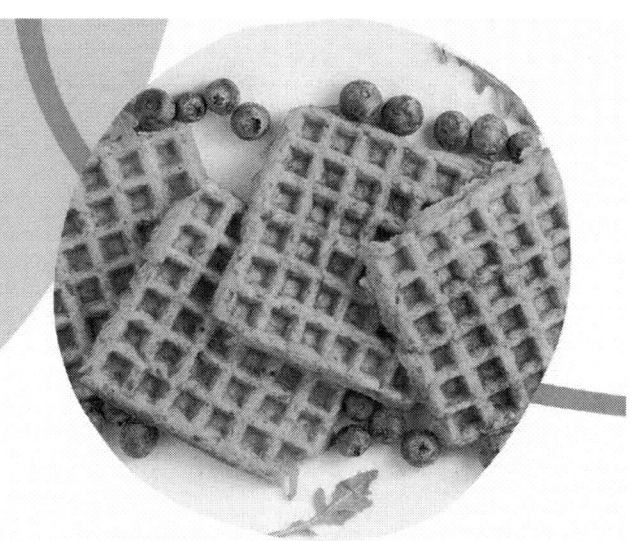

DIRECTIONS

1. Begin by preparing the blueberry sauce. For this, you need to take a saucepan and place it on a medium-high flame.
2. Add in the water, lemon zest, lemon juice, blueberries, honey, cloves, and molasses. Mix well and let it come to a boil.
3. Reduce the flame to low and cover the saucepan with a lid. Simmer the sauce for around 5 minutes. The sauce should be slightly thickened by now. Set aside and let it stay covered to keep warm.
4. Take another large saucepan and fill it with water. Place it over a high flame. Bring the water to a boil.
5. While the water boils, add in the diced sweet potato. Once the water boils again, reduce the flame to medium and cook for around 10 minutes.
6. Once done, transfer the boiled sweet potato to the blender and blend until it turns into a smooth paste. Set aside.
7. Take a large glass mixing bowl and add in the all-purpose flour, whole-wheat flour, cornmeal, salt, baking powder, cinnamon, ginger, and baking powder. Mix well.

SWEET POTATO BREAKFAST WAFFLES

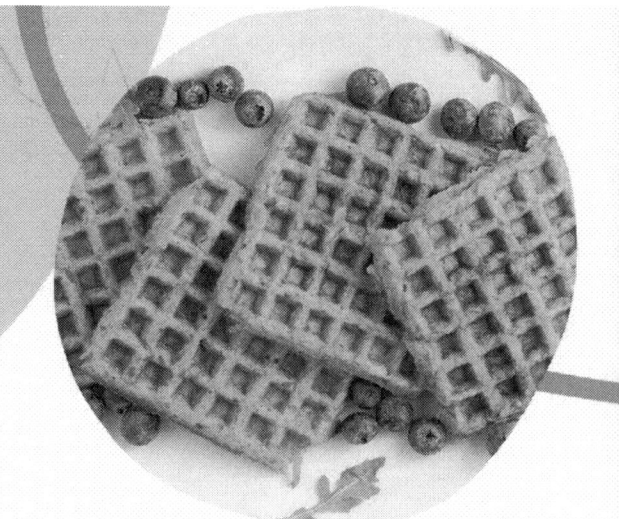

DIRECTIONS

8. Now add in the blended sweet potato, soy milk, molasses, and olive oil. Mix until all ingredients are well combined.
9. Take another bowl and add in the egg whites; use an electric mixer to beat until soft peaks form. Use the mixer on high speed to get the right texture.
10. Now gradually transfer the beaten egg into the flour mixture and fold it with a spatula. Make sure that the beaten eggs are completely incorporated.
11. Take a waffle iron and let it heat through. Use a measuring cup to scoop out the prepared batter and drop it onto the waffle iron. Cook for about 3-4 minutes, then transfer onto a serving platter. Repeat the process with the remaining batter.
12. Once done, top with the prepared blueberry sauce.
13. Serve!

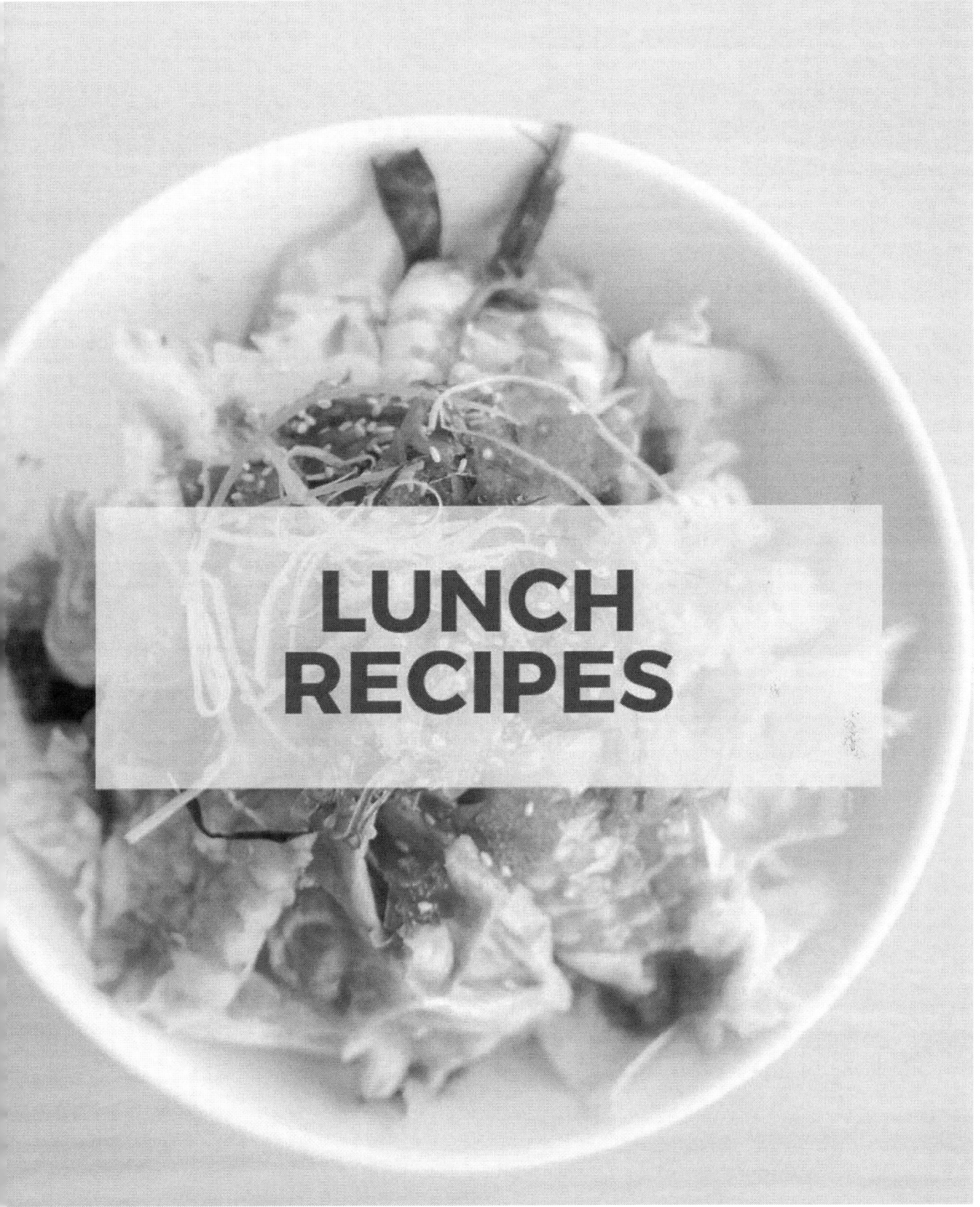

LUNCH RECIPES

ASIAN-STYLE PORK TENDERLOIN

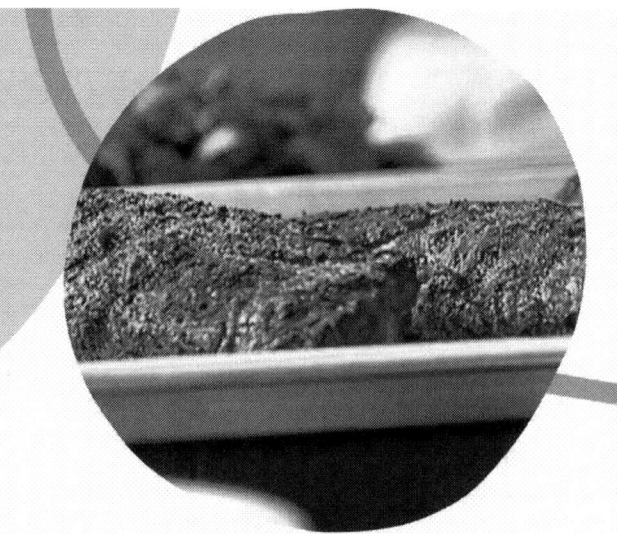

GENERAL INFO

Serving size: 1
Servings per recipe: 4
Calories: 176 calories per serving

INGREDIENTS

Sesame seeds – 2 tablespoons
Ground coriander – 1 teaspoon
Cayenne pepper – ⅛ teaspoon
Celery seed – ⅛ teaspoon
Onion (minced) – ½ teaspoon
Ground cumin – ¼ teaspoon
Ground cinnamon – ⅛ teaspoon
Sesame oil – 1 tablespoon
Pork tenderloin – 1 pound

NUTRITION INFO

Protein – 24 g
Sodium – 61 mg
Carbohydrates – 1 g
Fat – 8 g

ASIAN-STYLE PORK TENDERLOIN

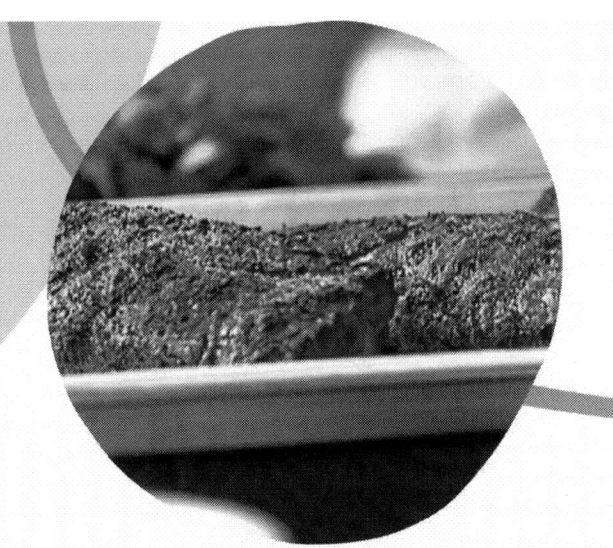

DIRECTIONS

1. Begin by slicing the pork tenderloins into 4 equal portions.
2. Preheat the oven by setting the temperature to 400 degrees Fahrenheit.
3. Take a baking dish and lightly coat it with nonstick coating spray.
4. Take a cast iron pan and place it over a low flame. Add in the sesame seeds and arrange them in a single layer. Roast the seeds for around 2 minutes, stirring continuously. Make sure to not burn the seeds or they may lose their taste. Remove from the flame and set it aside to cool.
5. Take a glass bowl and add in the coriander, celery seed, cayenne pepper, minced onion, cinnamon, cumin, toasted sesame seeds, and sesame oil. Mix well.
6. Place the sliced pork tenderloins into the greased baking dish and coat it with a prepared spice mixture on both sides.
7. Place the baking dish into the preheated oven and bake for around 15 minutes.
8. Once done, transfer onto a serving platter and serve right away!

BAKED CHICKEN WITH HERBED WILD RICE

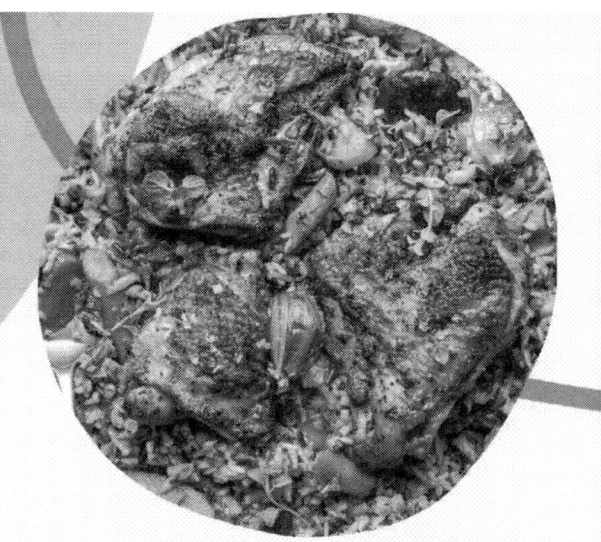

GENERAL INFO

Serving size: 1 ½ cups
Servings per recipe: 6
Calories: 313 calories per serving
Total time: 1 hour 20 minutes

INGREDIENTS

Chicken breast halves (skinless and boneless) – 1 pound
Celery (chopped) – 1 ½ cups
Whole pearl onions – 1 ½ cups
Fresh tarragon – 1 teaspoon
Chicken broth (unsalted) – 2 cups
Long-grain white rice (uncooked) – ¾ cup
Wild rice (uncooked) – ¾ cup
Dry white wine – 1 ½ cups

NUTRITION INFO

Protein – 23 g
Sodium – 104 mg
Carbohydrates – 38 g
Fat – 3 g

BAKED CHICKEN WITH HERBED WILD RICE

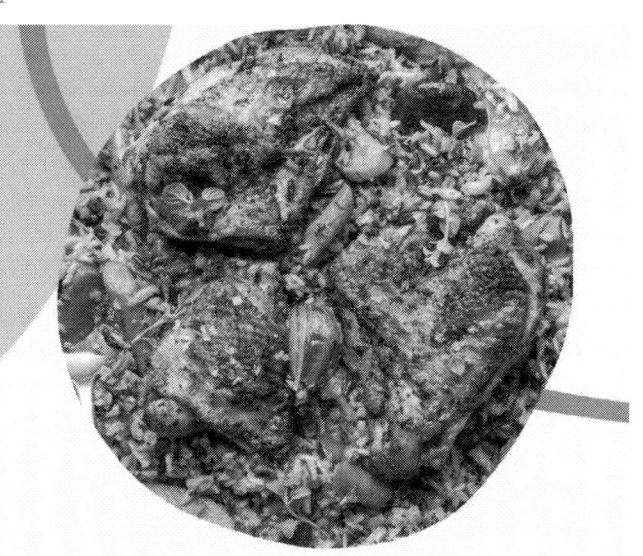

DIRECTIONS

1. Begin by preheating the oven by setting the temperature to 300 degrees Fahrenheit.
2. Cut the chicken breasts into pieces measuring about 1 inch each and set them aside.
3. Take a nonstick pan and add in the chicken pieces, celery, tarragon, and onion. Mix well.
4. Also, pour a cup of chicken broth into the same and cook for around 10 minutes. Make sure the vegetables are nicely cooked and tender. Set aside until it cools.
5. Take a baking dish and add in the remaining chicken broth, rice, and wine. Set aside and let it soak for about 30 minutes.
6. Add the cooked vegetables and chicken to the rice mixture and give it a nice stir.
7. Cover the baking dish with a foil sheet and place it in the preheated oven for about an hour.
8. Once done, transfer onto a serving plate and serve immediately.

BAKED COD TOPPED WITH CAPERS AND LEMON

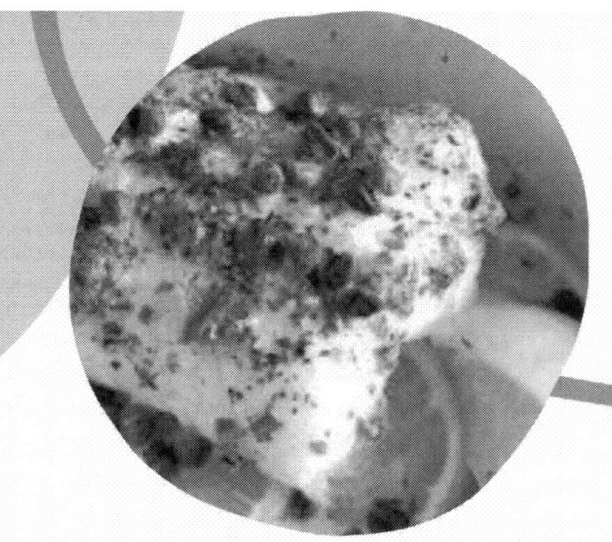

GENERAL INFO

Serving size: 1
Servings per recipe: 4
Calories: 159 calories per serving
Total time: minutes

INGREDIENTS

Cod fillets – 4 (6 ounces each)
Lemon – 1
Low-sodium bouillon granules (chicken-flavored) – 1 teaspoon
Hot tap water – 1 cup
Butter (softened) – 1 tablespoon
All-purpose flour – 1 tablespoon
Capers (drained and rinsed) – 4 teaspoons

NUTRITION INFO

Protein – 30 g
Sodium – 294 mg
Carbohydrates – 3 g
Fat – 3 g

BAKED COD TOPPED WITH CAPERS AND LEMON

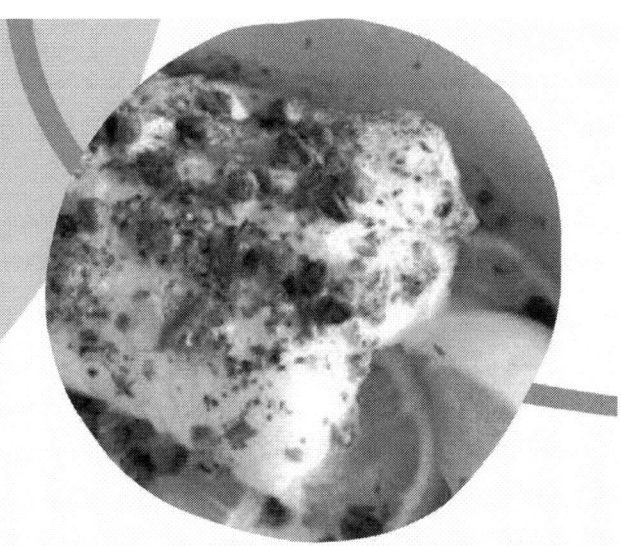

DIRECTIONS

1. Begin by preheating the oven by setting the temperature to 350 degrees Fahrenheit.
2. Take 4 aluminum foil sheets and spray each with nonstick cooking spray.
3. Place 1 cod fillet into each of the foil squares.
4. Cut a lemon in half and squeeze half of the lemon juice on the fish. Cut the remaining half into slices and place it over the fillet. Seal all ends of the aluminum foil and set aside. Repeat the process with the remaining fillets.
5. Place the fish parcels into the preheated oven and cook for around 20 minutes.
6. While the fish cooks, take a small glass mixing bowl and add in the bouillon granules and hot water. Stir well and set aside. Make sure the granules are completely dissolved.
7. Take another bowl and add in the flour and butter. Mix until well combined.
8. Transfer it to a heavy-bottom saucepan and place it over a medium flame. Stir well until the butter is melted.
9. Add the bouillon mixture to the butter and flour mixture and stir until the sauce begins to thicken.
10. Add in the capers and cook for a couple of minutes.
11. Take the fish out of the oven and transfer the baked cod onto a serving platter.
12. Pour the prepared sauce onto the fish and serve!

BAKED RED SAUCE MACARONI

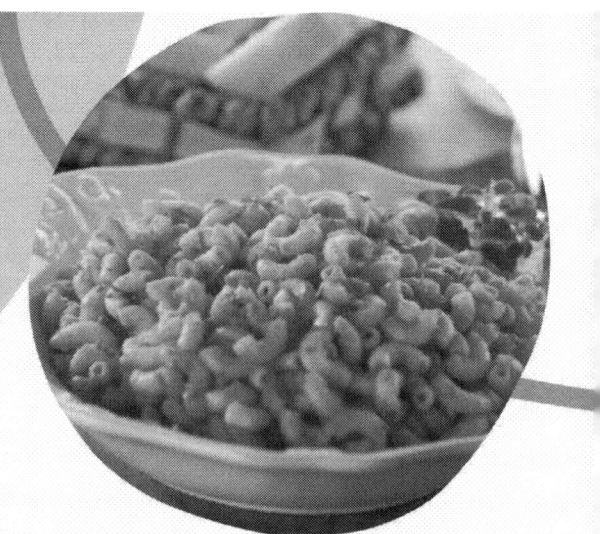

GENERAL INFO

Serving size: 1 cup
Servings per recipe: 6
Calories: 269 calories per serving
Total time: 55 minutes

INGREDIENTS

Ground beef (extra-lean) – ½ pound
Onion (diced) – 1 small
Elbow macaroni (whole-wheat) – 1 box
Spaghetti sauce (reduced-sodium) – 1 jar (15 ounces)
Parmesan cheese – 6 tablespoons

NUTRITION INFO

Protein – 15 g
Sodium – 125 mg
Carbohydrates – 32 g
Fat – 9 g

BAKED RED SAUCE MACARONI

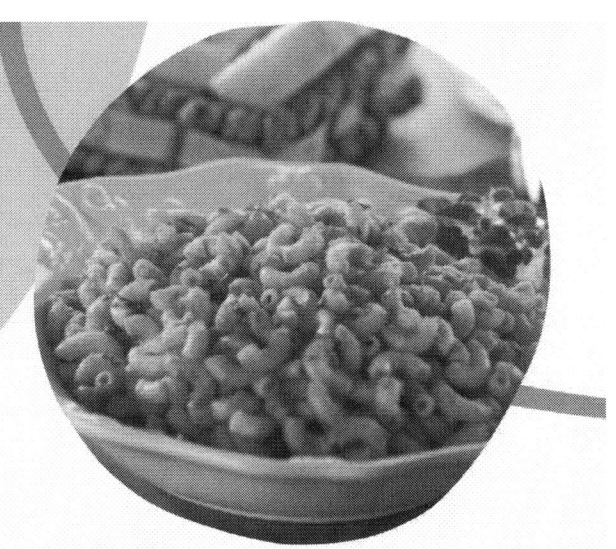

DIRECTIONS

1. Begin by preheating the oven by setting the temperature to 350 degrees Fahrenheit.
2. Take a baking dish and lightly grease it with cooking spray.
3. Take a cast iron pan and place it on a medium-high flame. Add in the onion and ground beef; cook until the onion becomes translucent and the meat is nicely browned. Drain the excess fat and set it aside.
4. Take a large stockpot and fill it halfway with water. Once the water begins to boil, add in the pasta and cook as per package directions. Drain the pasta into a colander and set aside.
5. Transfer the cooked pasta into the onion and meat mixture. Also, add in the spaghetti sauce. Mix until all ingredients are well incorporated.
6. Transfer the pasta and meat into the greased baking dish and place it in the preheated oven.
7. Bake the pasta and meat for around 35 minutes. Once done, take it out of the oven.
8. Finish by sprinkling parmesan cheese on top. Transfer onto a serving platter and serve hot!

BAKED SALMON TOPPED WITH ASIAN MARINADE

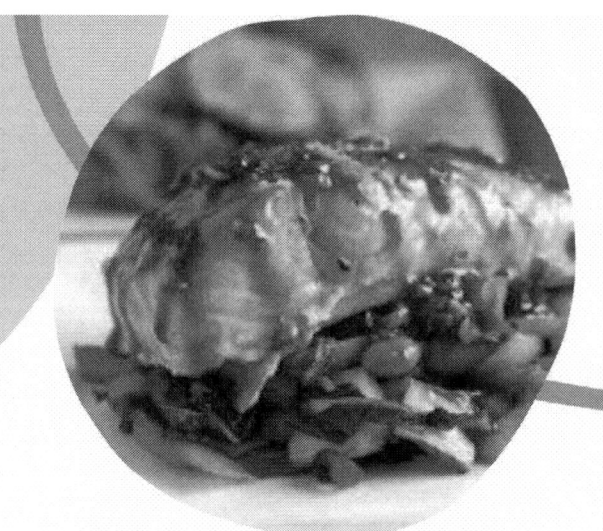

GENERAL INFO

Serving size: 1
Servings per recipe: 2
Calories: 247 calories per serving

INGREDIENTS

Pineapple juice – ½ cup
Garlic (minced) – 2 cloves
Soy sauce (low-sodium) – 1 teaspoon
Ground ginger – ¼ teaspoon
Salmon fillets – 2 (4 ounces each)
Sesame oil – ¼ teaspoon
Black pepper (freshly ground) – as per taste
Mixed fruit (pineapple, mango, and papaya) – 1 cup

NUTRITION INFO

Protein – 27 g
Sodium – 192 mg
Carbohydrates – 19 g
Fat – 7 g

BAKED SALMON TOPPED WITH ASIAN MARINADE

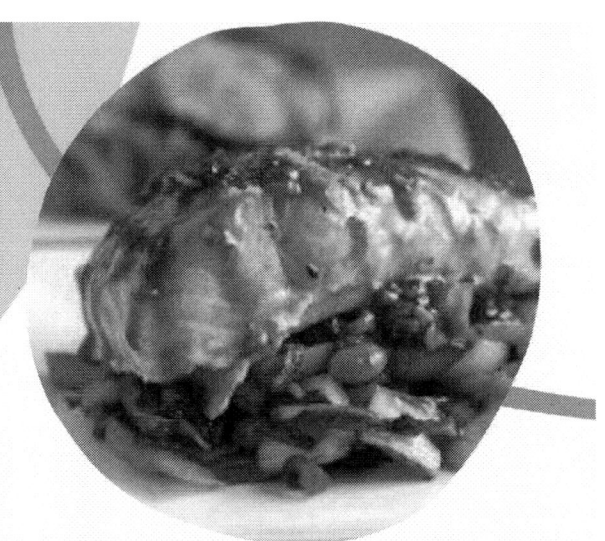

DIRECTIONS

1. Take a small bowl and add in the garlic, pineapple juice, ginger, and soy sauce. Mix until well combined.
2. Take a baking dish and place the salmon fillets into the same. Top the fillets with the pineapple juice mixture and place it in the refrigerator to marinate for around an hour. Flip the fish halfway through.
3. While the fillet is marinating, set the temperature of the oven to 375 degrees Fahrenheit.
4. Take 2 aluminum sheets and place them on a flat surface. Grease them lightly with cooking spray. Place 1 marinated fillet on each of the sheets.
5. Top each fillet is with an equal amount of sesame oil and diced fruit. Also, top with freshly ground black pepper. Take the edges of the foil and seal it into a parcel.
6. Place the parcel into the preheated oven and baked for around 10 minutes; flip over and bake for another 10 minutes.
7. Transfer onto a serving platter and serve right away!

BRUSSELS SPROUTS WITH LEMON AND SHALLOTS

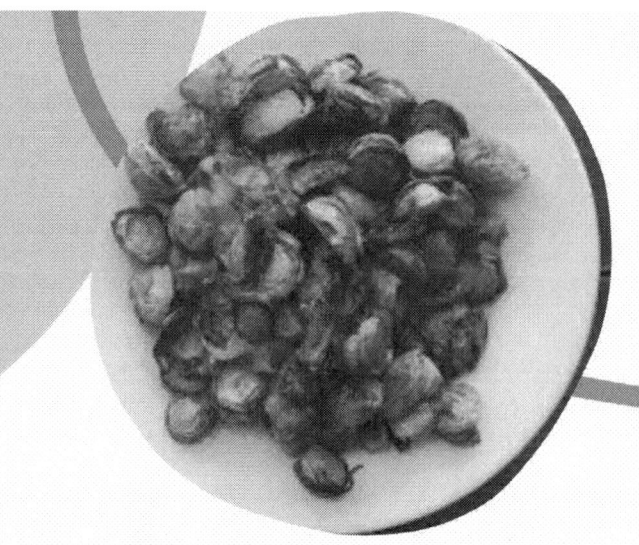

GENERAL INFO

Serving size: 1
Servings per recipe: 4
Calories: 104 calories per serving

INGREDIENTS

Olive oil (extra-virgin) – 3 teaspoons
Shallots (thinly sliced) – 3 small
Salt (divided) – ¼ teaspoon
Brussels sprouts – 1 pound
Vegetable stock (no salt added) – ½ cup
Lemon zest (finely grated) – ¼ teaspoon
Fresh lemon juice – 1 tablespoon
Black pepper (freshly ground) – ¼ teaspoon

NUTRITION INFO

Protein – 5 g
Sodium – 191 mg
Carbohydrates – 12 g
Fat – 4 g

BRUSSELS SPROUTS WITH LEMON AND SHALLOTS

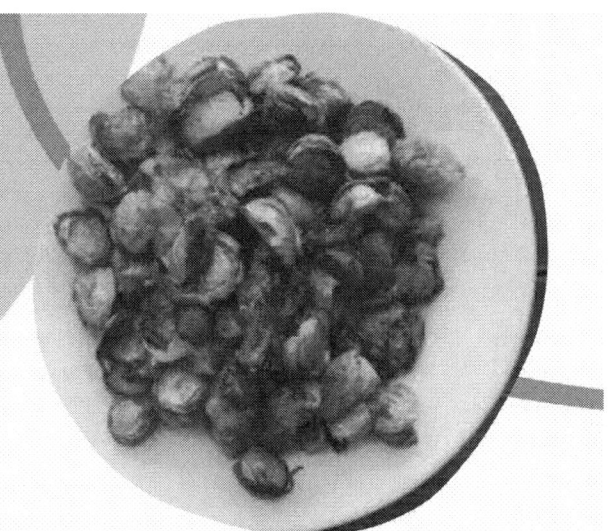

DIRECTIONS

1. Start by trimming the Brussels sprouts and cutting them into quarters.
2. Take a large cast-iron pan and place it on a medium-high flame. Pour in a couple of teaspoons of olive oil.
3. Add in the finely sliced shallots and keep stirring to sauté for around 6 minutes. Make sure the shallots are golden and not caramelized. Sprinkle ⅛ teaspoon of salt over the shallots and stir. Once done, transfer the shallots into a small bowl and set aside.
4. Return the pan to the flame and add in the remaining teaspoon of olive oil.
5. Toss in the quartered Brussels sprouts and cook for about 4 minutes. Keep stirring to prevent them from caramelizing.
6. Pour in the vegetable stock and let it simmer. Cook for about 6 minutes or until the Brussels sprouts are tender.
7. Return the sautéed shallots to the Brussels sprouts and vegetable stock. Add in the lemon juice and lemon zest. Stir well.
8. Finish by seasoning the Brussels sprouts with ⅛ teaspoon of freshly ground pepper. Mix well. Serve and enjoy!

CHICKEN BURRITOS

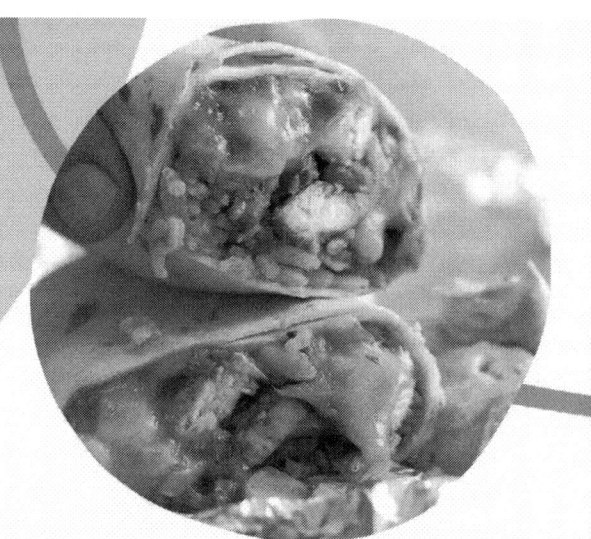

GENERAL INFO

Serving size: 1
Servings per recipe: 4
Calories: 286 calories per serving
Total time: 40 minutes

INGREDIENTS

Oil – 1 teaspoon
Red bell pepper (finely chopped) – 1
Jalapeno pepper (seeded and finely chopped) – 1
Celery ribs (chopped) – 2
Yellow onion (finely chopped) – 1
Cumin seed – 2 tablespoons
Grape tomatoes – 2 cups
Fresh oregano – 2 tablespoons
Garlic (chopped) – 2 cloves
Chicken breasts (cooked) – 8 ounces
Tortillas (whole-wheat) – 4 (10-inch diameter)
Canned black beans (drained and rinsed) – ½ cup
Green cabbage (shredded) – 2 cups

NUTRITION INFO

Protein – 20 g
Sodium – 382 mg
Carbohydrates – 38 g
Fat – 6 g

CHICKEN BURRITOS

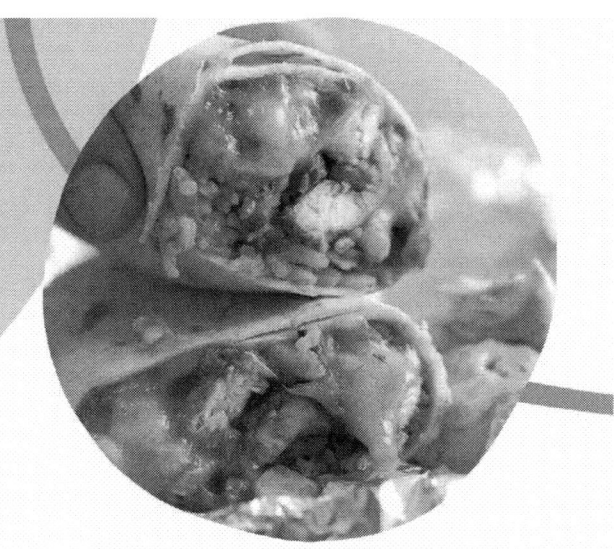

DIRECTIONS

1. Take a large nonstick skillet and place it on a medium-high flame.
2. Pour in the oil and let it heat through. Toss in the onion, celery, cumin, and pepper. Sauté for around 15 minutes. Continue stirring to prevent the ingredients from sticking to the bottom.
3. Now add in the tomatoes, garlic, and oregano and continue to cook for another 10 minutes.
4. Transfer the ingredients to a blender and blend into a smooth puree-like consistency.
5. Place the cooked chicken breasts onto a plate and use a fork to pull the chicken apart.
6. Place the tortillas on a flat surface and begin assembling. Top each tortilla with an equal amount of pulled chicken. Top the chicken with cabbage, beans, and the sauce.
7. Roll the tortillas into burritos. Enjoy and serve right away!

CHICKEN SALAD (GRILLED) WITH BUTTERMILK DRESSING

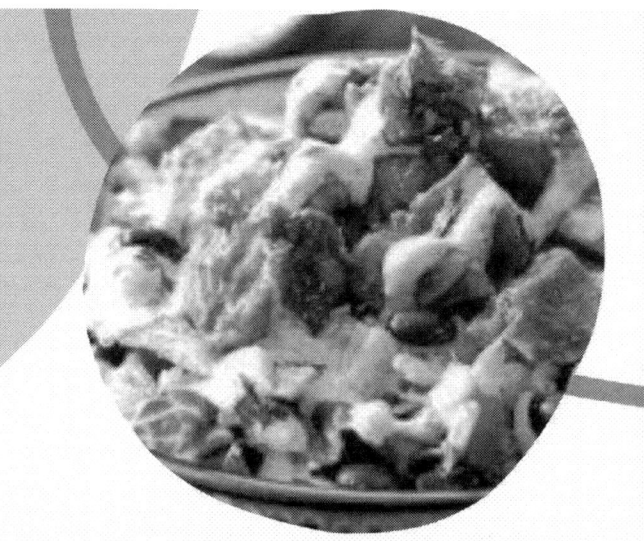

GENERAL INFO

Serving size: 1
Servings per recipe: 4
Calories: 222 calories per serving
Total time: 25 minutes

INGREDIENTS

For dressing:
Mayonnaise (fat-free) – 1/3 cup
Buttermilk (low-fat) – ¼ cup
Fresh dill (finely chopped) – 2 tablespoons
Garlic (minced) – 1 teaspoon
Black pepper (cracked) – as per taste

For salad:
Chicken breasts (boneless and skinless) – 4
Olive oil (extra-virgin) – 2 teaspoons
Salad greens (torn) – 8 cups
Red bell pepper (sliced) – 1
Sweet onion (sliced) – ½

NUTRITION INFO

Protein – 28 g
Sodium – 264 mg
Carbohydrates – 14 g
Fat – 6 g

CHICKEN SALAD (GRILLED) WITH BUTTERMILK DRESSING

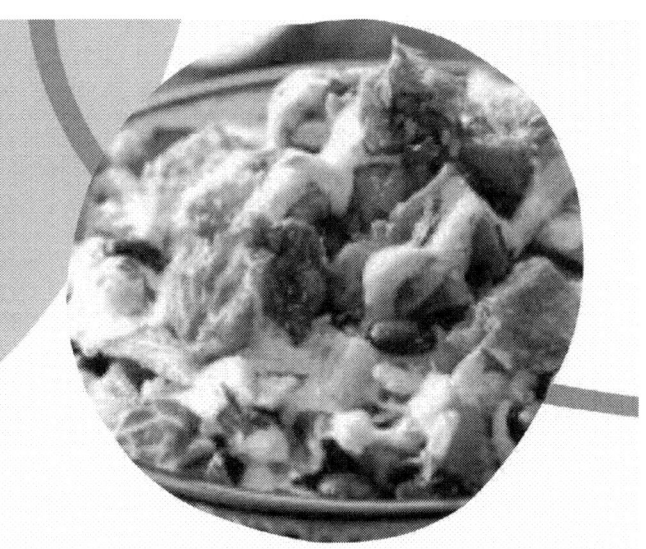

DIRECTIONS

1. Begin by taking a small bowl and adding in the buttermilk, mayonnaise, garlic, black pepper, and dill. Use a whisk to mix the ingredients well and transfer into a glass bowl. Cover it with a lid. Place the dressing in the refrigerator.
2. Prepare the charcoal grill and light the fire. Take the grill rack and lightly grease it with cooking spray. Place the greased rack 6 inches over the fire.
3. Place the chicken breasts on a shallow dish and brush them generously with olive oil. Place the chicken breasts onto the grill.
4. Grill the chicken breasts for 5 minutes; flip over and cook for another 5 minutes.
5. Once done, transfer the grilled chicken breasts to a chopping block for 5 minutes. Once the chicken is done resting, cut it into thin slices.
6. Take a large mixing bowl and add in the salad greens, onion, and bell pepper. Drizzle ¾ of the buttermilk dressing. Toss until all veggies are evenly coated.
7. Transfer about 2 cups of salad on each of the plates and place the sliced chicken on top.
8. Finish with a final drizzle of buttermilk dressing.
9. Serve right away!

CHICKEN SALAD WITH BALSAMIC VINAIGRETTE & PINEAPPLE

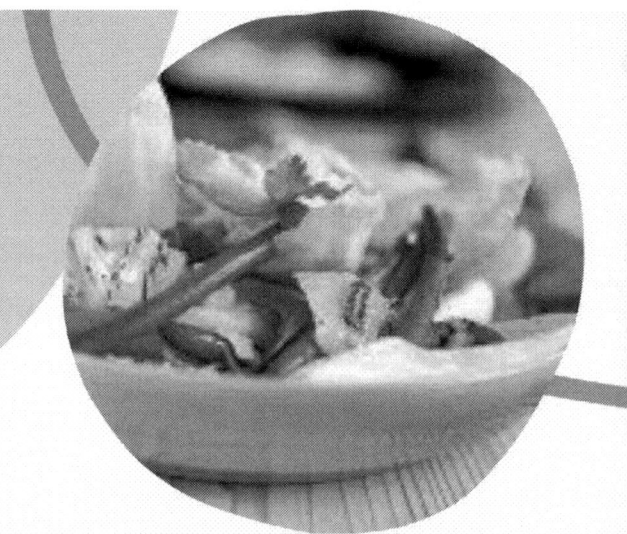

GENERAL INFO

Serving size: 2 cups
Servings per recipe: 8
Calories: 186 calories per serving
Total time: 15 minutes

NUTRITION INFO

Protein – 17 g
Sodium – 50 mg
Carbohydrates – 7 g
Fat – 10 g

INGREDIENTS

Chicken breasts (boneless and skinless) – 4
Olive oil – 1 tablespoon
Pineapple chunks (unsweetened) – 1 (8-ounce) can (save 2 tablespoons of juice)
Broccoli florets – 2 cups
Fresh baby spinach – 4 cups
Red onions (thinly sliced) – ½ cup

For vinaigrette:
Olive oil – ¼ cup
Balsamic vinegar – 2 tablespoons
Sugar – 2 teaspoons
Cinnamon (ground) – ¼ teaspoon

CHICKEN SALAD WITH BALSAMIC VINAIGRETTE & PINEAPPLE

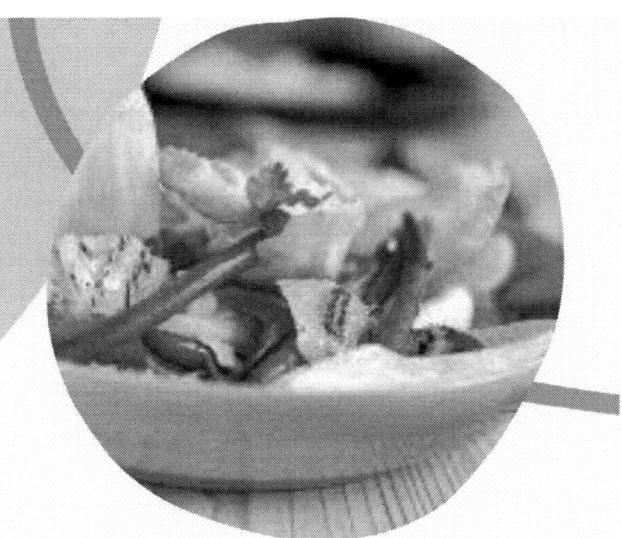

DIRECTIONS

1. Begin by cutting the chicken breasts into bite-sized cubes.
2. Take a large nonstick pan and place it on a medium flame. Pour in the olive oil and let it heat through.
3. Once the oil is hot, add in the chicken and sauté for around 10 minutes. Make sure the chicken is golden brown and slightly charred on the edges.
4. Take a large glass mixing bowl and add in the pineapple chunks, spinach, broccoli, onions, and chicken chunks. Toss well and set aside
5. To prepare the dressing, add the olive oil, reserved pineapple juice, vinegar, cinnamon, and sugar to a glass mixing bowl. Mix well to combine.
6. Pour the prepared dressing onto the chicken and veggies and toss until all ingredients are evenly coated.
7. Transfer onto a salad platter and serve!

CLAMS FETTUCCINE

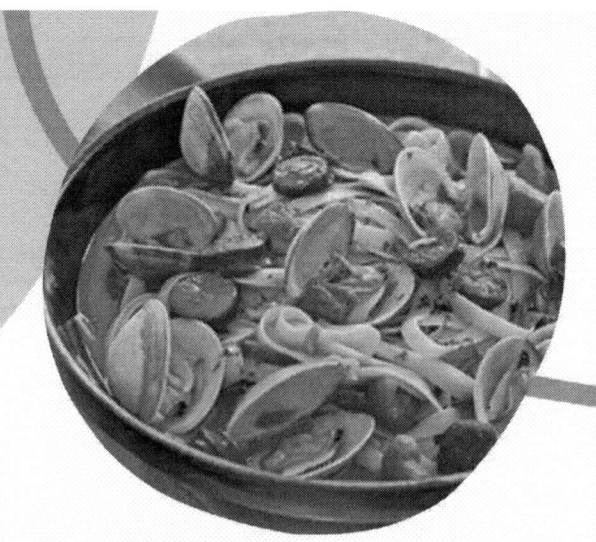

GENERAL INFO

Serving size: 1 ½ cups
Servings per recipe: 6
Calories: 316 calories per serving
Total time: 25 minutes

INGREDIENTS

Fettuccine (uncooked) – 10 ounces
Garlic (minced) – 2 tablespoons
Tomatoes – 2 large
Corn kernels – 2 cups
White wine – ½ cup
Olive oil – 1 tablespoon
Fresh basil (chopped) – 4 tablespoons
Clams (drained) – 2 cans
Salt – ¼ teaspoon
Black pepper (freshly ground) – as per taste

NUTRITION INFO

Protein – 18 g
Sodium – 147 mg
Carbohydrates – 52 g
Fat – 4 g

CLAMS FETTUCCINE

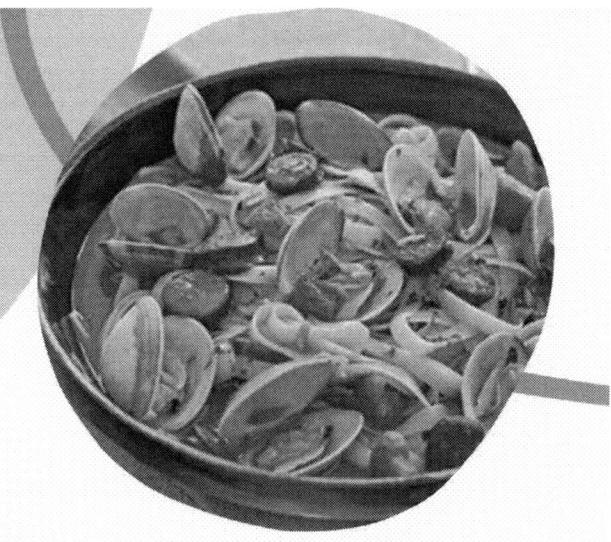

DIRECTIONS

1. Begin by seeding the tomatoes and cutting them into small chunks. Set aside.
2. Take a large stockpot and fill it halfway with water. Let it come to a boil.
3. Throw in the pasta and cook for around 8 minutes. Once done, drain it into a colander and set aside.
4. Take a large nonstick saucepan and add in the olive oil, garlic, corn, tomatoes, basil, and wine. Mix well and cover the pan with a lid. Keep stirring and let it come to a boil.
5. Once the sauce comes to a boil, reduce the flame and toss in the clams and cooked fettuccine.
6. Season the pasta with pepper and salt. Mix well.
7. Serve immediately.

CLASSIC CHICKEN QUESADILLAS

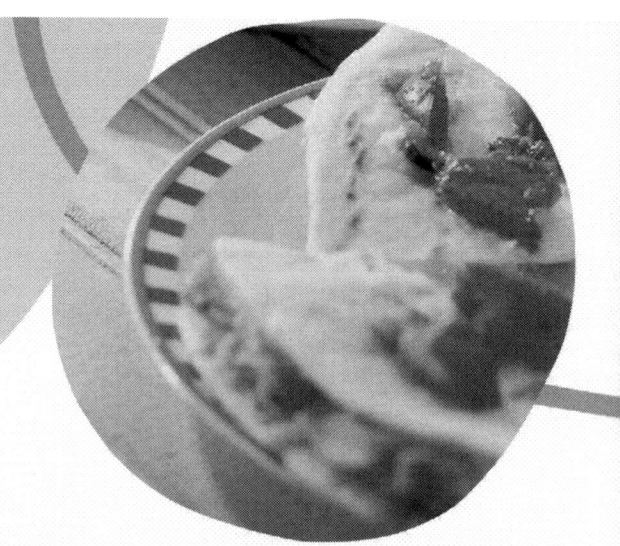

GENERAL INFO

Serving size: 1
Servings per recipe: 6
Calories: 298 calories per serving

INGREDIENTS

Chicken breasts (skinless and boneless) – 4
Onions (chopped) – 1 cup
Hot salsa – ½ cup
Fresh tomatoes (chopped) – 1 cup
Fresh cilantro (chopped) – 1 cup
Tortillas (whole-wheat) – 6
Shredded cheddar cheese (reduced-fat) – 1 cup

NUTRITION INFO

Protein – 27 g
Sodium – 524 mg
Carbohydrates – 25 g
Fat – 10 g

CLASSIC CHICKEN QUESADILLAS

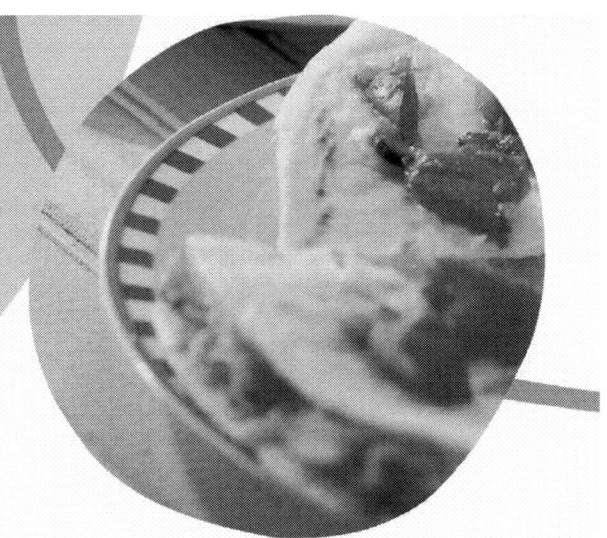

DIRECTIONS

1. Begin by preheating the oven by setting the temperature to 425 degrees Fahrenheit.
2. Take a baking dish and gently coat it with cooking spray.
3. Take the chicken breasts and cut them into bite-sized cubes. Set aside.
4. Take a large cast-iron pan and add in the onions and chicken. Sauté until the chicken is nicely cooked and the onions become translucent. This will take about 7 minutes. Remove from the flame and add in the tomato, cilantro, and salsa. Stir well to combine.
5. To assemble the quesadillas, place the tortillas on a flat surface and brush the edges with water.
6. Divide the prepared chicken and salsa mixture equally and place it in the center of the tortillas. Top the chicken mixture with shredded cheddar cheese.
7. Fold a tortilla in half and press the edges to seal it. Repeat the same process with the rest of the tortillas.
8. Place the tortillas on a cookie sheet and place the cookie sheet onto a baking dish.
9. Use cooking spray to coat the tortillas.
10. Place the baking dish into the preheated oven and bake for around 7 minutes.
11. Once done, cut each tortilla in half. Serve right away!

CREAMY POLENTA WITH VEGGIES

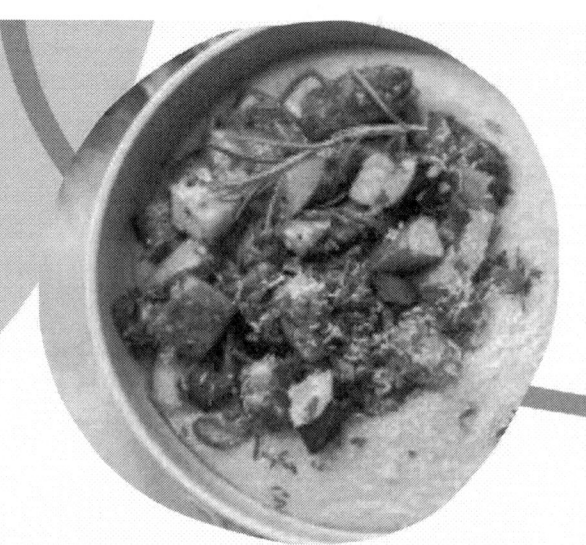

GENERAL INFO

Serving size: 1
Servings per recipe: 4
Calories: 178 calories per serving
Total time: 50 minutes

INGREDIENTS

Cornmeal/polenta (coarsely ground) – 1 cup
Water – 4 cups
Garlic (chopped) – 1 teaspoon
Fresh mushrooms (sliced) – 1 cup
Onions (sliced) – 1 cup
Broccoli florets – 1 cup
Zucchini (sliced) – 1 cup
Parmesan cheese (grated) – 2 tablespoons
Fresh oregano (chopped) – as per taste

NUTRITION INFO

Protein – 6 g
Sodium – 55 mg
Carbohydrates – 34 g
Fat – 1 g

CREAMY POLENTA WITH VEGGIES

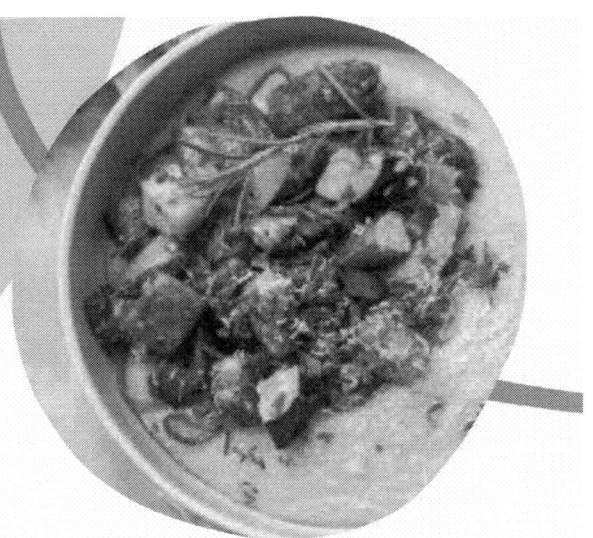

DIRECTIONS

1. Begin by preheating the oven by setting the temperature to 350 degrees Fahrenheit.
2. Take a glass baking dish and lightly coat it with cooking spray.
3. Add polenta, garlic, and water to a mixing bowl and mix well. Transfer into the baking dish.
4. Place the baking dish into the oven and bake for around 40 minutes.
5. While the polenta cooks, place the nonstick pan on a medium flame. Coat the pan with cooking spray.
6. Once the pan is hot, add in the onions and mushrooms. Sauté until the veggies are nicely tender; this will take around 5 minutes.
7. Place a steamer on a medium-high flame and add the zucchini and broccoli to the steamer basket. Cover the lid and steam for around 3 minutes. The veggies should be tender yet crisp.
8. Once the polenta is done, take the baking dish out of the oven and top it with steamed zucchini and broccoli.
9. Finish by sprinkling the veggies with herbs and parmesan cheese.
10. Serve right away!

FLANK STEAK AND ROASTED CORN SALAD

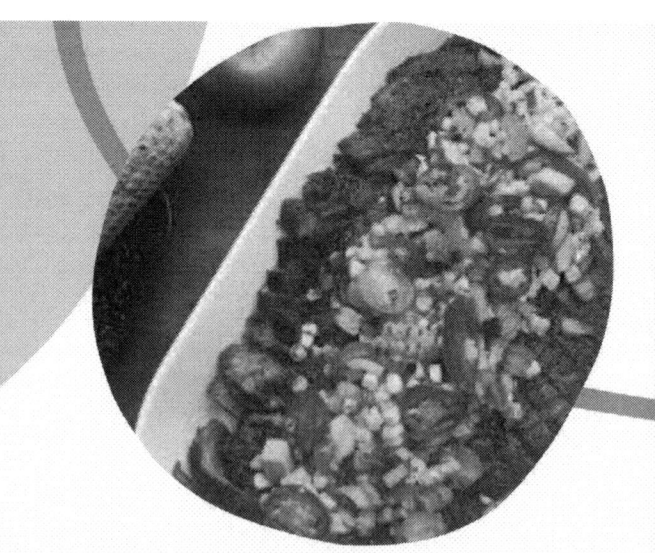

GENERAL INFO

Serving size: 1
Servings per recipe: 6
Calories: 295 calories per serving
Total time: 30 minutes

NUTRITION INFO

Protein – 21 g
Sodium – 249 mg
Carbohydrates – 37 g
Fat – 9 g

INGREDIENTS

Fresh corn kernels – 3 cups
Water – ½ cup
Fresh lime juice – 2 tablespoons
Red bell pepper (chopped) – 2 tablespoons
Olive oil (extra-virgin) – 2 tablespoons
Salt – ½ teaspoon
Black pepper (freshly ground) – ½ teaspoon
Fresh cilantro (chopped) – ¼ cup
Ground cumin – 1 tablespoon
Dried oregano – 2 teaspoons
Red pepper flakes – ¼ teaspoon
Flank steak – ¾ pound
Romaine lettuce – 1 large head
Cherry tomatoes (halved) – 4 cups
Red onion (thinly sliced) – ¾ cup
Black beans (cooked) – 1 ½ cups

FLANK STEAK AND ROASTED CORN SALAD

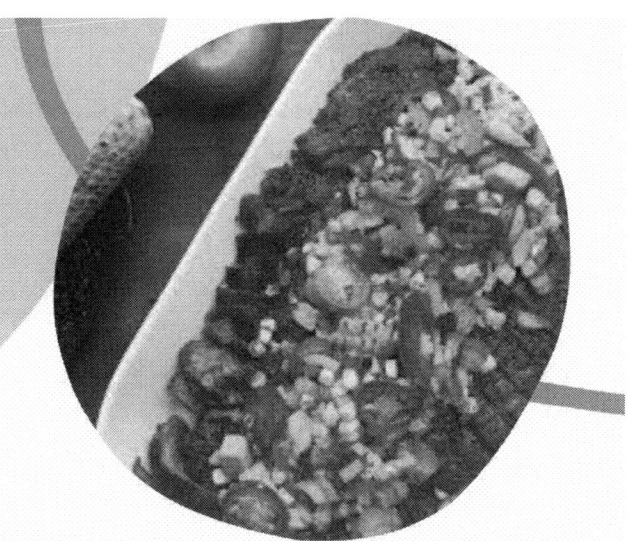

DIRECTIONS

1. Begin by trimming the romaine lettuce and tearing it into bite-sized pieces.
2. Place a large cast-iron pan on a medium-high flame and add in the corn. Dry roast for about 5 minutes. Continue stirring to prevent the kernels from burning. Once done, set aside.
3. Take a blender and add in the water, bell pepper, lime juice, and a cup of roasted corn. Blend into a smooth puree-like consistency.
4. Now add the olive oil, cilantro, ¼ teaspoon of salt, and ¼ teaspoon of black pepper to the blender. Blend again until you have a smooth puree-like consistency. Set aside.
5. Prepare a charcoal grill by starting a fire. Take the grill rack and lightly coat it with the cooking spray. Place the grill rack 6 inches from the fire.
6. Take a small mixing bowl and add in the cumin, red pepper flakes, oregano, remaining salt, and remaining black pepper. Mix well.
7. Place the steak in a shallow dish and sprinkle the prepared spice mix. Rub it evenly on both sides.

FLANK STEAK AND ROASTED CORN SALAD

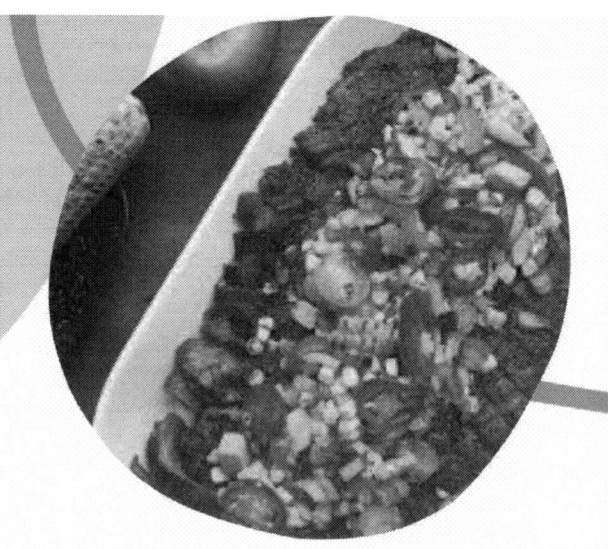

DIRECTIONS

8. Place the steak on the grill rack and cook for 5 minutes; flip over and cook for another 5 minutes. Once done, set aside to cool for at least 5 minutes.
9. Slice the steak into ¼-inch slices and set aside.
10. Take a large mixing bowl and add in the lettuce, onion, tomatoes, 3 cups of roasted corn, and black beans. Toss well to combine the ingredients.
11. Pour the prepared vinaigrette over the veggies and mix gently until all ingredients are evenly coated.
12. Serve the prepared salad on the plates and serve each plate with sliced steak.

An Appeal from the Publisher

Hello wonderful reader!

We hope you are enjoying this book.

We wanted to let you know that you have made an impact on many lives by reading this book.

Just to give you a brief introduction: We are a small publishing company with a team of 8 writers and 2 editors.

Most of our employees come from financially weaker section and our company is the only means they support their families. This is our way of giving back to the society.

We don't have the giant advertising budgets that many other publishers and businesses do online.

So, one way that you can really support our mission and our business is by leaving us a review on this book.

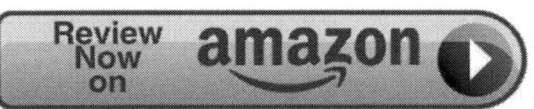

For a small company like us, getting reviews (especially on Amazon) means we can submit our books for advertising.

This means we can actually sell a few copies from time to time and make a bigger impact on the society as a whole. So, every review means a lot to us.

We can't THANK YOU enough for this!

PORK TENDERLOIN CURRY IN APPLE CIDER

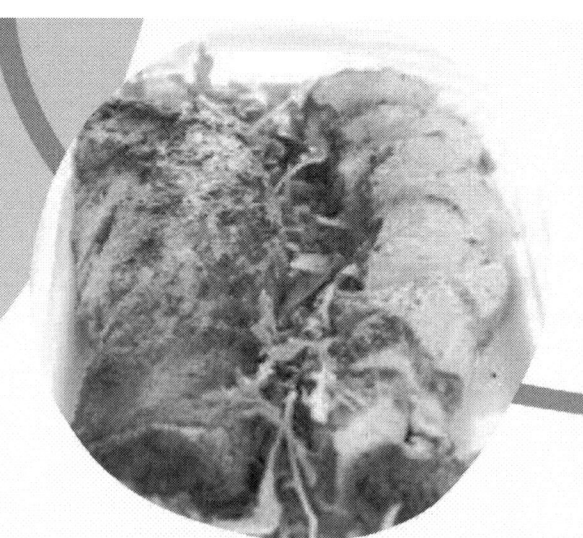

GENERAL INFO

Serving size: 1
Servings per recipe: 4
Calories: 270 calories per serving
Total time: 50 minutes

INGREDIENTS

Pork tenderloin – 16 ounces
Curry powder – 1 ½ tablespoons
Olive oil (extra-virgin) – 1 tablespoon
Yellow onions (chopped) – 2 medium
Apple cider – 2 cups
Tart apple – 1
Cornstarch – 1 tablespoon

NUTRITION INFO

Protein – 25 g
Sodium – 70 mg
Carbohydrates – 29 g
Fat – 6 g

PORK TENDERLOIN CURRY IN APPLE CIDER

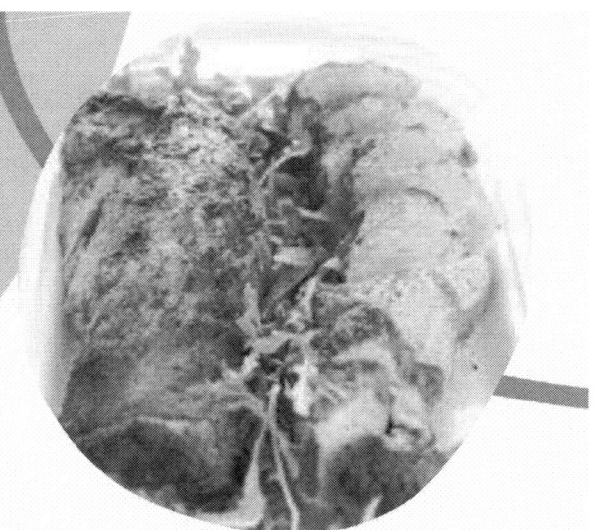

DIRECTIONS

1. Begin by cutting the pork tenderloin into 4 equal-sized pieces.
2. Take the tart apple; peel and remove the seeds. Cut the apple into bite-sized chunks.
3. Take a shallow dish and place the pork tenderloin into the same. Sprinkle the tenderloin pieces with curry powder and use your hands to coat the meat evenly. Set aside for around 15 minutes.
4. Take a cast-iron skillet and place it on a medium-high flame. Pour in the olive oil and let it heat through.
5. Add the pork tenderloin pieces to the skillet and cook for 7 minutes; flip over and cook for another 7 minutes.
6. Once done, put the pork onto a plate and set it aside.
7. Return the skillet to the flame and toss in the onions. Once the onions begin to caramelize, add the 1 ½ cups of apple cider. Reduce the flame and let the sauce simmer until it reduces to half.
8. Now add in the chopped tart apple, ½ cup of apple cider, and cornstarch. Give it a nice stir and let it simmer for about 2 minutes or until the sauce thickens.
9. Return the pork tenderloins to the sauce and cook for another 5 minutes on a low flame.
10. Once done, use a tong to place the pork tenderloins on a serving platter. Pour the prepared sauce over the meat.
11. Serve and enjoy!

STRIP STEAK WITH MUSHROOM WHISKEY SAUCE

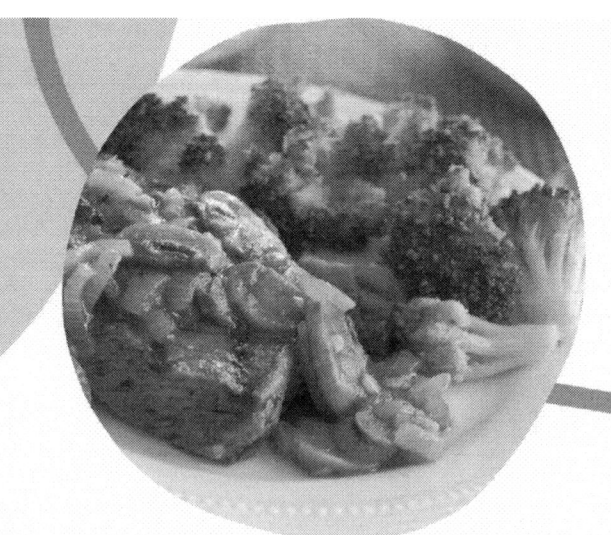

GENERAL INFO

Serving size: 1
Servings per recipe: 2
Calories: 330 calories per serving
Total time: 35 minutes

INGREDIENTS

New York strip steaks – 2
Margarine (trans-free) – 1 teaspoon
Garlic (chopped) – 3 cloves
Shiitake mushrooms (sliced) – 2 ounces
Button mushrooms – 2 ounces
Thyme – ¼ teaspoon
Rosemary – ¼ teaspoon
Whiskey – ¼ cup

NUTRITION INFO

Protein – 24 g
Sodium – 94 mg
Carbohydrates – 4 g
Fat – 17 g

STRIP STEAK WITH MUSHROOM WHISKEY SAUCE

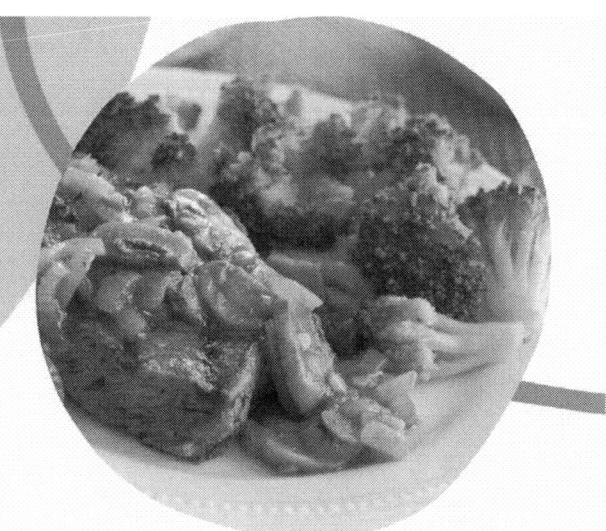

DIRECTIONS

1. Begin by preparing a fire in the charcoal grill.
2. Take the grill rack and coat it lightly with cooking spray. Place the grill rack about 6 inches above the fire.
3. Place the steak onto the grill and cook for around 10 minutes; flip over and cook for another 10 minutes.
4. Take a nonstick saucepan and place it on a medium flame. Add in the margarine and let it heat through. Add in the garlic, thyme, rosemary, and mushrooms. Sauté for around 2 minutes or until the mushrooms are tender.
5. Once done, remove the saucepan from the flame and pour in the whiskey. Cook for about a minute.
6. Place the steaks on a serving plate and top them with the whiskey sautéed mushrooms. Serve and enjoy!

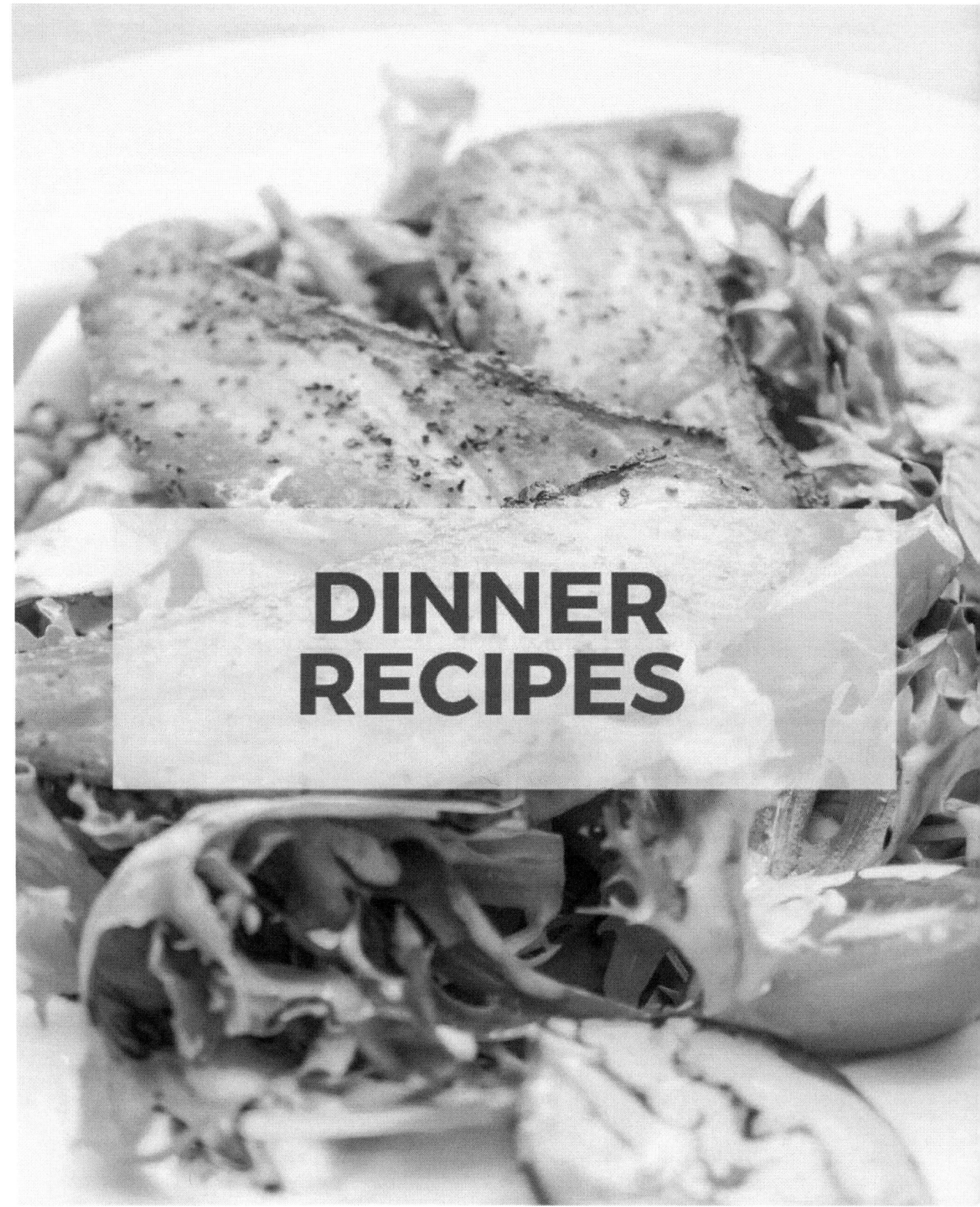

DINNER RECIPES

ASIAN-STYLE GRILLED SALMON

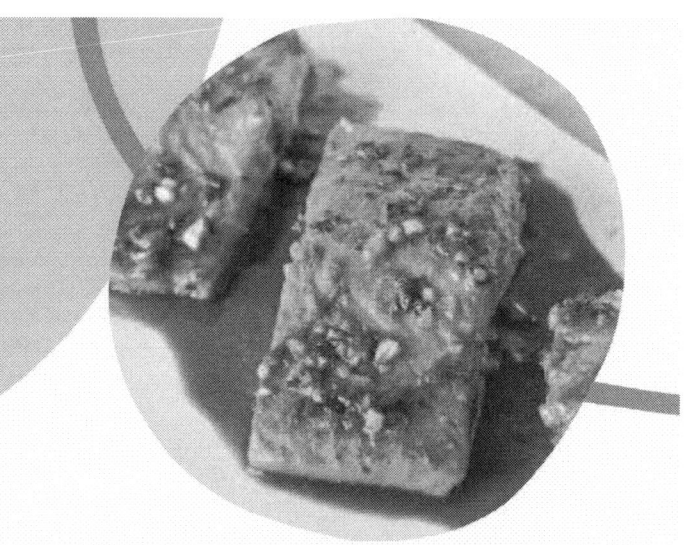

GENERAL INFO

Serving size: 1
Servings per recipe: 4
Calories: 185 calories per serving
Total time: 1 hour 15 minutes

INGREDIENTS

Sesame oil – 1 tablespoon
Soy sauce (reduced-sodium) – 1 tablespoon
Fresh ginger (minced) – 1 tablespoon
Rice wine vinegar – 1 tablespoon
Salmon fillets – 4

NUTRITION INFO

Protein – 26 g
Sodium – 113 mg
Carbohydrates – 1 g
Fat – 9 g

ASIAN-STYLE GRILLED SALMON

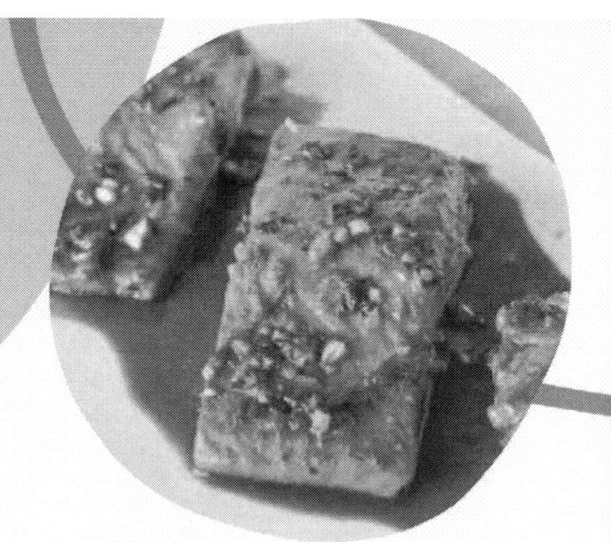

DIRECTIONS

1. Take a shallow dish and add in the sesame oil, ginger, vinegar, and soy sauce. Mix well to combine.
2. Place the salmon fillets in the dish and flip over to coat both sides. Place the marinated salmon into the fridge for around an hour. Flip after every 15 minutes.
3. Prepare the grill by lighting the fire and lightly coat the grill rack with oil. Make sure the temperature is medium-high.
4. Place the marinated fish fillets on the rack and cook for 5 minutes on each side. Make sure the fish is no longer pink.
5. Serve warm!

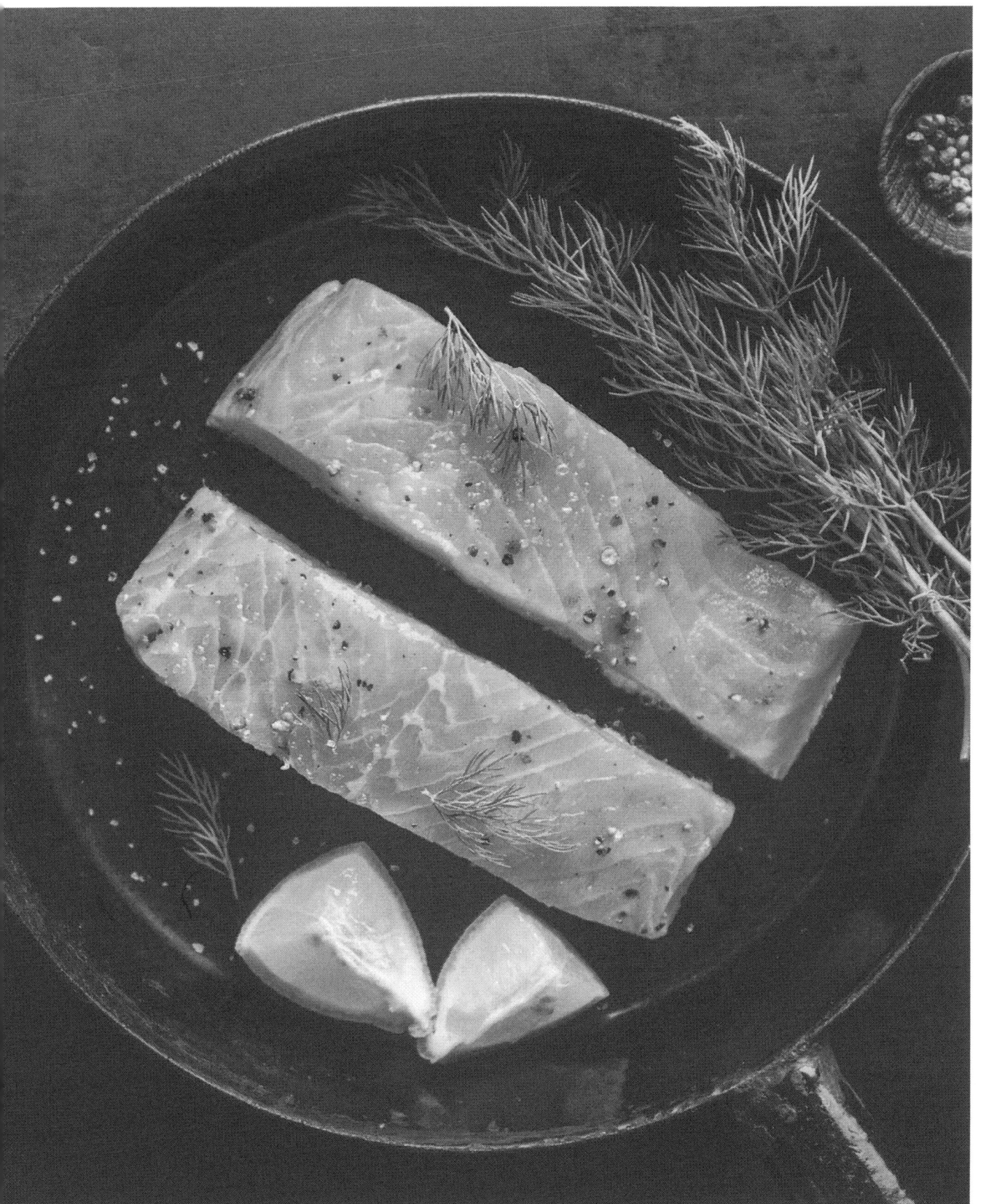

BAKED HERB-CRUSTED COD

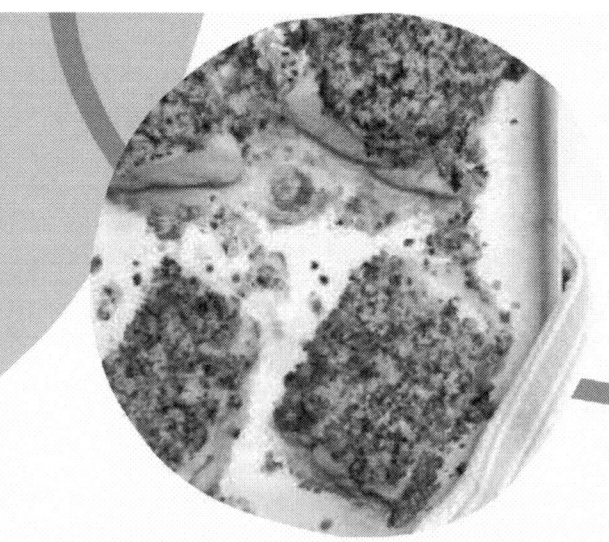

GENERAL INFO

Serving size: 1
Servings per recipe: 4
Calories: 150 calories per serving
Total time: 20 minutes

INGREDIENTS

Herb-flavored stuffing – ¾ cup
Cod fillets – 4
Honey – 2 tablespoons

NUTRITION INFO

Protein – 21 g
Sodium – 158 mg
Carbohydrates – 14 g
Fat – 1 g

BAKED HERB-CRUSTED COD

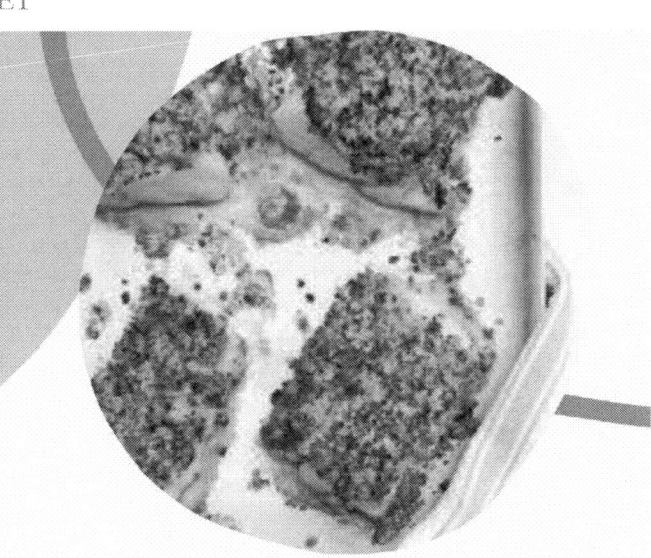

DIRECTIONS

1. Start by preheating the oven by setting the temperature to 375 degrees Fahrenheit.
2. Take a baking dish and coat it gently with cooking spray.
3. Take a zip-lock bag and add in the stuffing. Seal the bag and crush the stuffing until it is crumbly.
4. Place the fillets on a rack and brush them all with honey. Add one fillet to the zip-lock bag and coat it evenly with crumbly filling. Keep on a plate. Repeat the process with the remaining fillets.
5. Place the fillets into the prepared baking dish and place the dish into the preheated oven. Bake for 10 minutes.
6. Serve!

BARLEY AND TOMATO ROAST RISOTTO

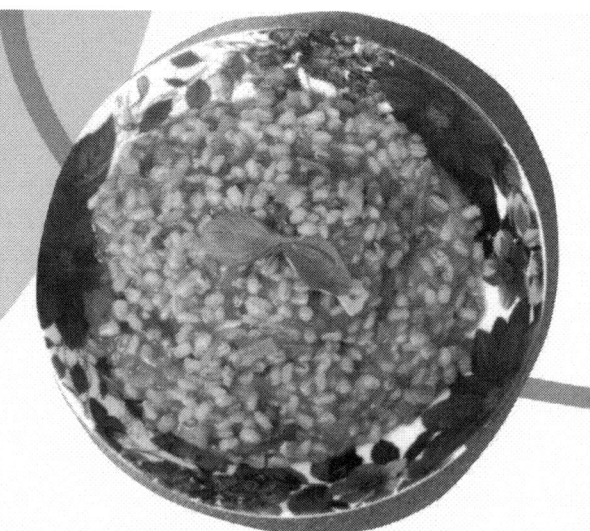

GENERAL INFO

Serving size: 1 ¼ cups
Servings per recipe: 8
Calories: 287 calories per serving
Total time: 1 hour 40 minutes

NUTRITION INFO

Protein – 11 g
Sodium – 288 mg
Carbohydrates – 45 g
Fat – 7 g

INGREDIENTS

Plum tomatoes – 10 large
Olive oil (extra-virgin) – 2 tablespoons
Salt – ½ teaspoon
Black pepper (freshly ground) – ½ teaspoon
Vegetable stock (low-sodium) – 4 cups
Water – 3 cups
Shallots (chopped) – 2
Dry white wine – ¼ cup
Pearl barley – 2 cups
Fresh basil (chopped) – 3 tablespoons
Fresh flat-leaf parsley (chopped) – 3 tablespoons
Fresh thyme (chopped) – 1 ½ tablespoons
Parmesan cheese (grated) – ½ cup

BARLEY AND TOMATO ROAST RISOTTO

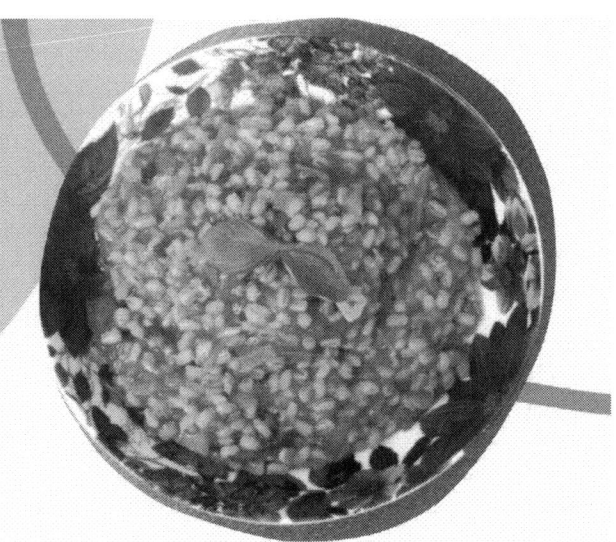

DIRECTIONS

1. Begin by preheating the oven by setting the temperature to 450 degrees Fahrenheit.
2. Take a large pan full of water and let it boil. Now add in the tomatoes and boil for about 5 minutes.
3. Take another bowl and fill it with cold water. Once the tomatoes are done, drop the tomatoes into the cold water.
4. Use a knife to peel the skin off the tomatoes and cut them into quarters. Set aside.
5. Take a nonstick baking dish and arrange the tomatoes in a single layer. Drizzle them with a tablespoon of olive oil and season them with ¼ teaspoon salt and pepper. Toss the tomatoes gently.
6. Place the baking sheet in the oven and roast for about 30 minutes. Once done, remove the baking sheet and keep 16 of the tomato wedges for garnishing.
7. Take a large cast-iron pan and place it on a high flame. Add in the water and vegetable stock and let it come to a boil. Reduce the flame to low and let it simmer.
8. Take another heavy saucepan and place it on a medium flame. Pour 1 tablespoon of olive oil and let it heat through.

BARLEY AND TOMATO ROAST RISOTTO

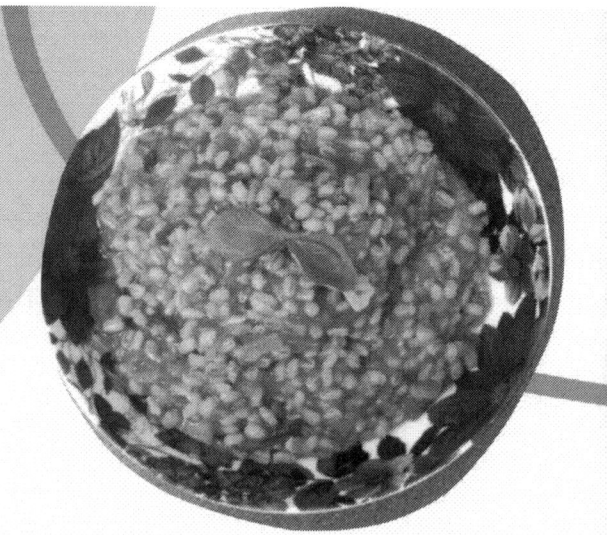

DIRECTIONS

10. Toss in the shallots and cook for about 3 minutes. Keep stirring to prevent the shallots from caramelizing.
11. Pour in the white wine to deglaze the pan and cook for about 3 minutes or until the liquid is almost evaporated.
12. Now add in the barley and stir well. Cook for about a minute. Stir in about ½ cup of vegetable stock and water mixture. Mix well and let it cook. Once the liquid is absorbed, add ½ cup more of the stock mixture and repeat the same until the mixture is finished. This will take about 50 minutes.
13. Once the barley is done cooking, turn off the flame and add in the chopped basil, roasted tomatoes, grated cheese, thyme, and parsley. Fold them gently.
14. Season the barley with the remaining pepper and salt. Mix until all ingredients are well combined.
15. Transfer the risotto into a serving bowl and garnish with basil leaves and reserved roasted tomatoes.
16. Serve right away!

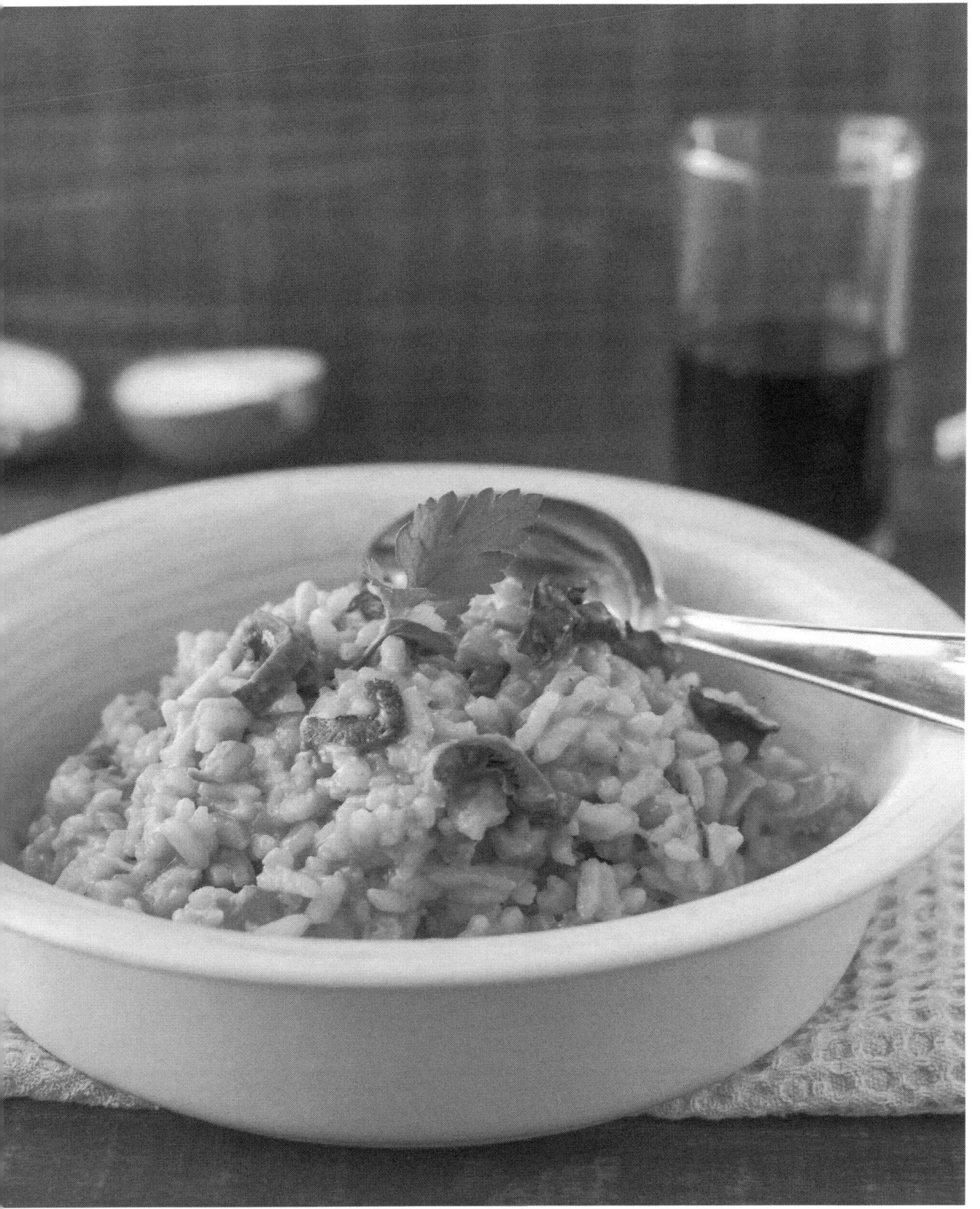

BLACK-EYED CREOLE-STYLE PEAS

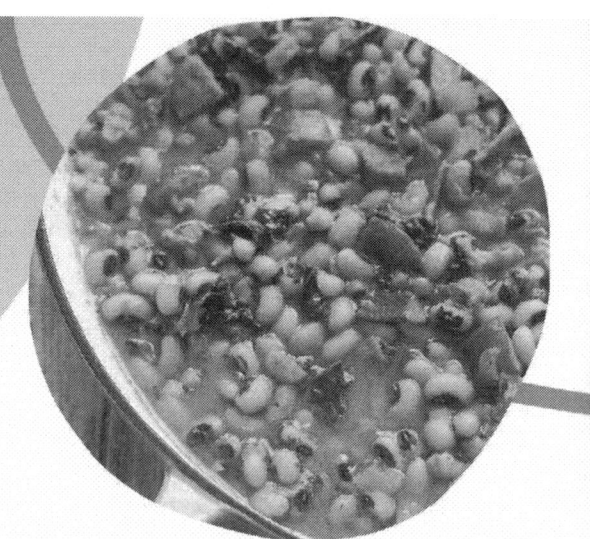

GENERAL INFO

Serving size: 1
Servings per recipe: 8
Calories: 168 calories per serving
Total time: 3 hours 15 minutes

INGREDIENTS

Water – 3 cups
Black-eyed peas – 2 cups dried
Low-sodium bouillon granules – 1 teaspoon
Unsalted canned tomatoes (crushed) – 2 cups
Onion (finely chopped) – 1 large
Celery (finely chopped) – 2 stalks
Garlic (minced) – 3 teaspoons
Dry mustard – ½ teaspoon
Ground ginger – ¼ teaspoon
Cayenne pepper – ¼ teaspoon
Bay leaf – 1
Parsley (chopped) – ½ cup

NUTRITION INFO

Protein – 11 g
Sodium – 50 mg
Carbohydrates – 31 g
Fat – 1 g

BLACK-EYED CREOLE-STYLE PEAS

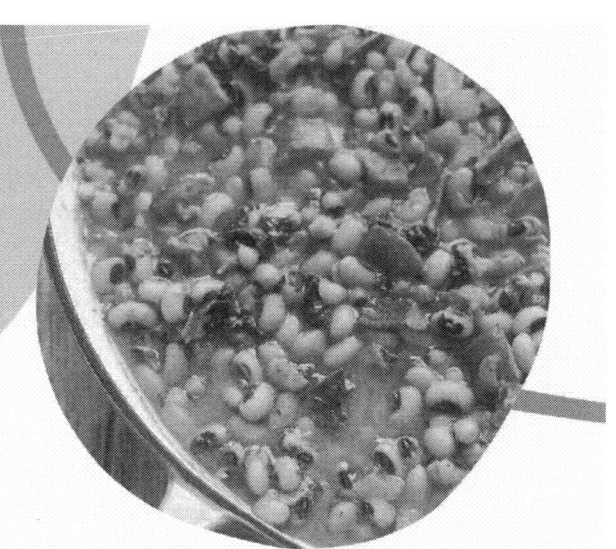

DIRECTIONS

1. Begin by taking a medium-sized saucepan and placing it over a high flame.
2. Pour 2 cups of water into the pan and also add in the black-eyed peas. Let it boil for about 2 minutes.
3. Once it begins to boil, cover the pan with a lid. Remove from the flame and set it aside for at least an hour.
4. Use a colander to drain excess water from the beans and return the drained peas to the pan.
5. Pour in the remaining 1 cup water into the saucepan and also add in the bouillon granules, onion, tomatoes, garlic, celery, cayenne pepper, bay leaf, ginger, and mustard. Give a nice stir.
6. Reduce the flame to low and cook for around 2 hours. Add more water if required.
7. Once done, get rid of the bay leaf and stir again.
8. Transfer into a serving bowl and finish by topping with parsley.
9. Serve and enjoy!

CHICKEN ASPARAGUS PENNE

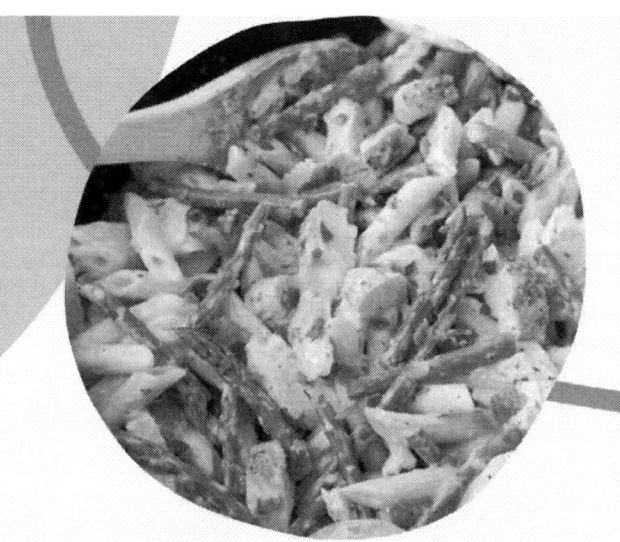

GENERAL INFO

Serving size: 1
Servings per recipe: 2
Calories: 433 calories per serving
Total time: 30 minutes

INGREDIENTS

Penne pasta (whole-grain) – 1 ½ cups
Asparagus – 1 cup, cut into 1-inch pieces
Chicken breasts (boneless and skinless) – 6 ounces, cut into 1-inch cubes
Garlic (minced) – 2 cloves
Tomatoes including juice (diced) – 1 (14.5 ounces) can
Dried oregano – 2 teaspoons
Soft goat cheese (crumbled) – 1 tablespoon
Parmesan cheese – 1 tablespoon

NUTRITION INFO

Protein – 34 g
Sodium – 140 mg
Carbohydrates – 54 g
Fat – 9 g

CHICKEN ASPARAGUS PENNE

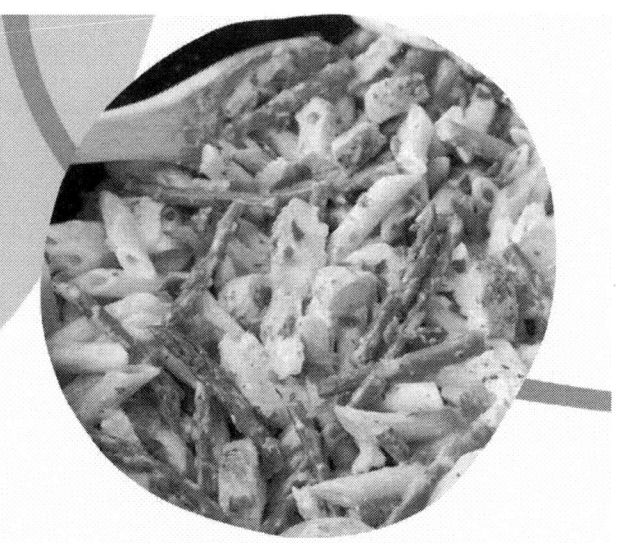

DIRECTIONS

1. Begin by cutting the asparagus into pieces measuring about an inch each. Also, cut the chicken breasts into 1-inch cubes.
2. Take a large stockpot and fill it with water. Let it come to a boil.
3. Once the water begins to boil, add in the pasta and cook as per package instructions. This will normally take about 10-12 minutes.
4. Once the pasta is al dente, drain into a colander and set aside.
5. Take a steamer and fill the steamer pot with water up to 1 inch in height. Add the cut asparagus to the steamer basket and place it over the pot once the water comes to a boil. Cover with a lid and steam for around 3 minutes.
6. While the asparagus steams, take a large nonstick pan and place it on a medium-high flame. Grease it lightly with cooking spray.
7. Add the garlic and chicken to the pan and sauté for about 7 minutes. The chicken should be golden brown.
8. Add in the tomatoes along with the juice and oregano and cook for another 1 minute. Stir well and remove from the flame.
9. Transfer the cooked pasta into a large glass mixing bowl along with the steamed asparagus and prepared chicken and tomato mixture. Also, add in the crumbled goat cheese and give a nice toss. Make sure all ingredients are well combined.
10. Serve on pasta plates topped with a generous sprinkle of parmesan cheese.
11. Enjoy!

EASY BEEF BRISKET

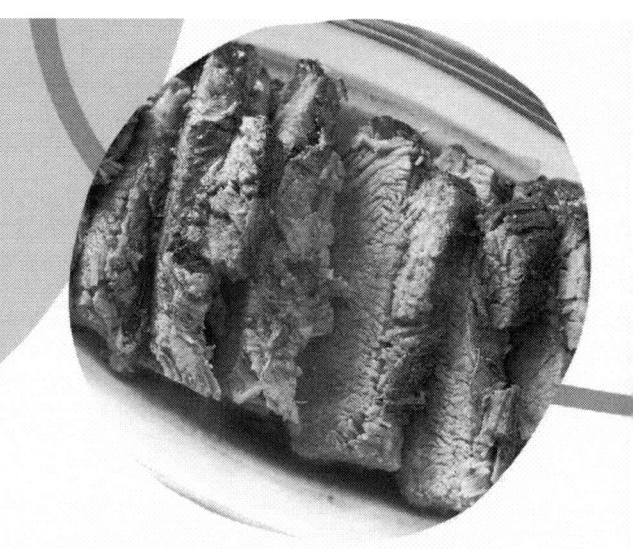

GENERAL INFO

Serving size: 1
Servings per recipe: 8
Calories: 229 calories per serving
Total time: 3 hours 50 minutes

INGREDIENTS

Olive oil – 1 tablespoon
Beef brisket – 2 ½ pounds
Black pepper (coarsely ground) – as per taste
Onions (chopped) – 1 ½ cups
Garlic (peel and smash) – 4 cloves
Dried thyme – 1 teaspoon
Tomatoes and liquid (no salt added) – 1 can (14.5 ounces)
Red wine vinegar – ¼ cup
Beef stock (low-sodium) – 1 cup

NUTRITION INFO

Protein – 31 g
Sodium – 184 mg
Carbohydrates – 6 g
Fat – 9 g

EASY BEEF BRISKET

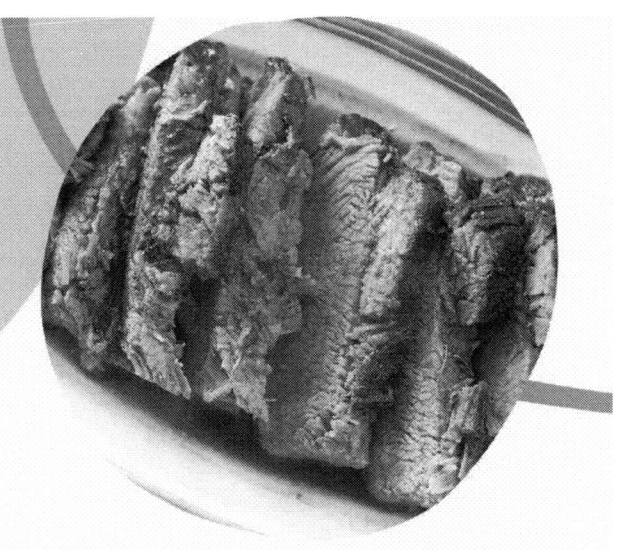

DIRECTIONS

1. Begin by trimming the fat off the beef brisket. Cut the brisket into 8 equal-sized pieces.
2. Preheat the oven by setting the temperature to 350 degrees Fahrenheit.
3. Place the brisket pieces in a shallow dish and sprinkle with coarsely ground pepper. Make sure the brisket is evenly coated.
4. Take a large-sized Dutch oven and place it on a medium-high flame. Pour in a tablespoon of oil and let it heat through.
5. Add the seasoned brisket pieces to the Dutch oven and cook until the meat turns dark brown on each side. This will take about 6-8 minutes. Turn every 2 minutes to prevent the meat from burning.
6. Once done, transfer the brisket onto a plate and set it aside.
7. Add the onion to the Dutch oven and sauté until it begins to caramelize. Also, add in the thyme and garlic and sauté for around a minute.
8. Now add in the tomatoes and the juice, beef stock, and vinegar. Mix well and let it come to a boil.
9. Return the sautéed beef brisket to the Dutch oven and cook with tomatoes and stock mixture for about 3 ½ hours or until the beef is tender.
10. Serve hot!

EASY BEEF STROGANOFF

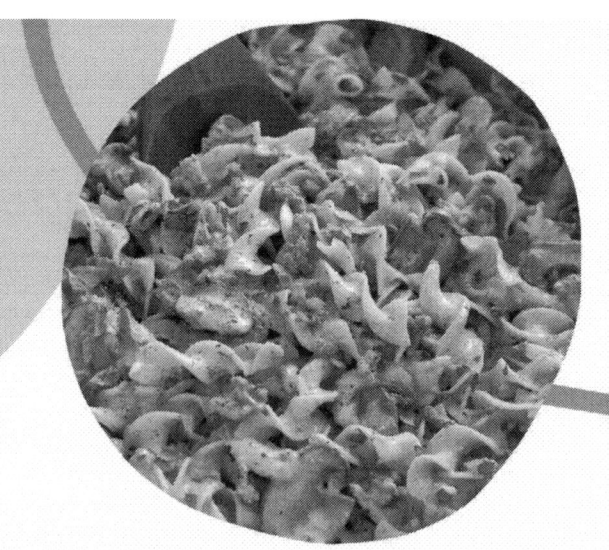

GENERAL INFO

Serving size: 2 ½ cups
Servings per recipe: 4
Calories: 273 calories per serving
Total time: 40 minutes

INGREDIENTS

Onion (chopped) – ½ cup
Beef round steak (boneless) – ½ pound
Yolkless egg noodles (uncooked) – 4 cups
Cream of mushroom soup (fat-free and undiluted) – ½ can
Water – ½ cup
All-purpose flour – 1 tablespoon
Paprika – ½ teaspoon
Sour cream (fat-free) – ½ cup

NUTRITION INFO

Protein – 20 g
Sodium – 193 mg
Carbohydrates – 37 g
Fat – 5 g

EASY BEEF STROGANOFF

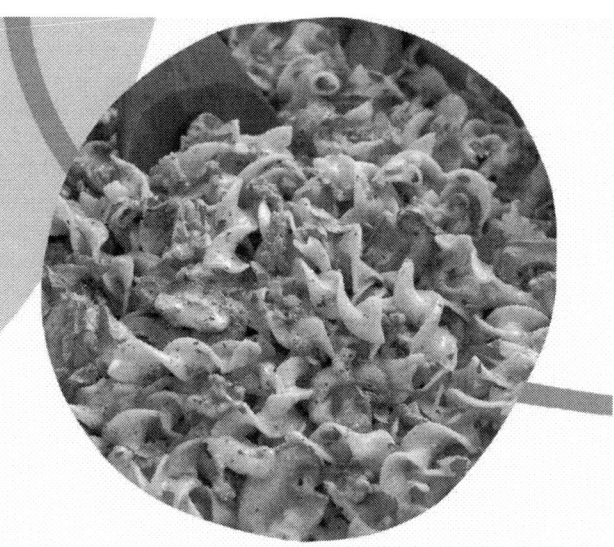

DIRECTIONS

1. Begin by cutting the beef round steak into slices measuring about ¾ inch each. Make sure that you remove all the fat.
2. Take a large cast-iron pan and place it on a medium flame. Add in the onions and sauté until they become translucent. This will take about 5 minutes.
3. Add in the beef and cook for 5 more minutes. Make sure the edges are browned and tender to touch. Drain any excess fat and set aside.
4. Take a large pot and fill it more than halfway. Place the pot on a high flame and let the water come to a boil.
5. Add noodles to the boiling water and cook for around 12 minutes or as per package instructions. Once done, drain into a colander and set aside.
6. Take a nonstick saucepan and place it on a medium flame. Add in the cream of mushroom soup, flour, and water; stir well and cook for around 5 minutes or until the sauce thickens.
7. Transfer the soup mixture to the beef and mixture; cook on a medium flame until the mixture is heated through. Add in the paprika and stir well. Remove from the flame.
8. Now add in the sour cream and stir to combine well.
9. To serve, place noodles on the plate and top with the soup and beef mixture.
10. Enjoy warm!

GARLIC AND BROCCOLI RIGATONI

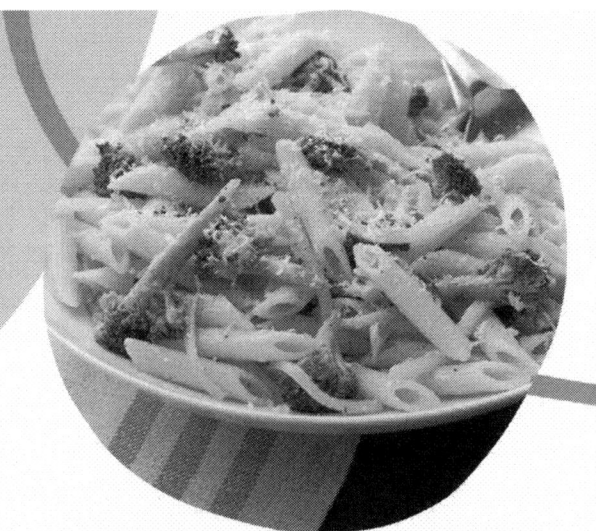

GENERAL INFO

Serving size: 2 cups
Servings per recipe: 2
Calories: 348 calories per serving
Total time: 25 minutes

INGREDIENTS

Rigatoni (whole-wheat) – 1/3 pound
Broccoli florets – 2 cups
Parmesan cheese – 2 tablespoons
Olive oil – 2 teaspoons
Garlic (minced) – 2 teaspoons
Black pepper (freshly ground) – as per taste

NUTRITION INFO

Protein – 16 g
Sodium – 106 mg
Carbohydrates – 53 g
Fat – 8 g

GARLIC AND BROCCOLI RIGATONI

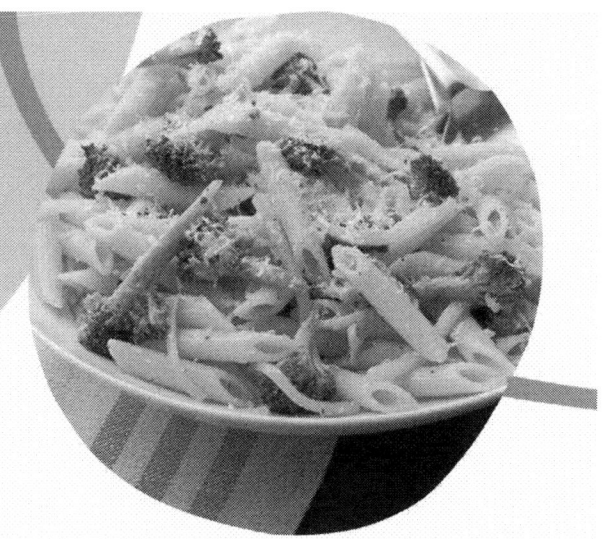

DIRECTIONS

1. Take a large pot and place it over a high flame. Fill it more than halfway and let it come to a boil.
2. Toss the pasta into the boiling water and cook it on high for around 12 minutes or as per package instructions.
3. While the pasta cooks, take a steamer and add the broccoli to the steamer basket. Fill the steamer pot with 2 cups of water. Cover the steamer basket with a lid and steam for around 10 minutes.
4. Once the pasta is cooked, drain it in a colander and set aside.
5. Take a large glass mixing bowl and add in the steamed broccoli and cooked pasta.
6. Also, add in the parmesan cheese, garlic, and olive oil. Generously season with freshly ground black pepper. Toss well until all ingredients are well combined.
7. Serve right away!

SPICED CHIPOTLE SHRIMP

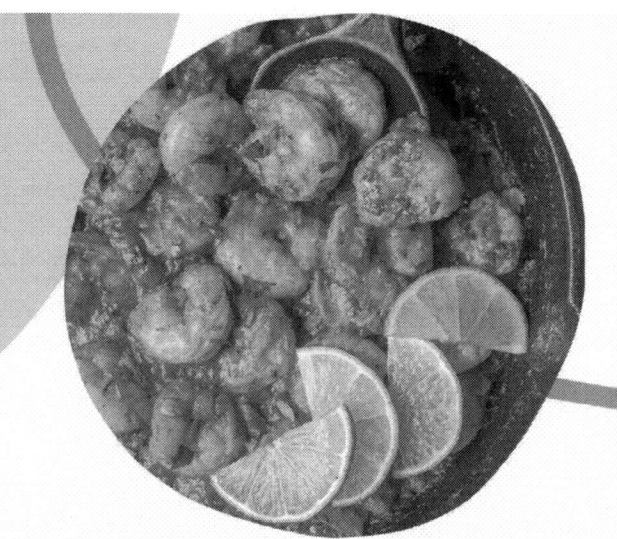

GENERAL INFO

Serving size: 1
Servings per recipe: 4
Calories: 109 calories per serving
Total time: 45 minutes

INGREDIENTS

Shrimp (uncooked; peeled and deveined) – 1 pound
Tomato paste – 2 tablespoons
Water – 1 ½ teaspoons
Olive oil (extra-virgin) – ½ teaspoon
Garlic (minced) – ½ teaspoon
Chipotle chili powder – ½ teaspoon
Fresh oregano (chopped) – ½ teaspoon

NUTRITION INFO

Protein – 23 g
Sodium – 139 mg
Carbohydrates – 2 g
Fat – 1 g

SPICED CHIPOTLE SHRIMP

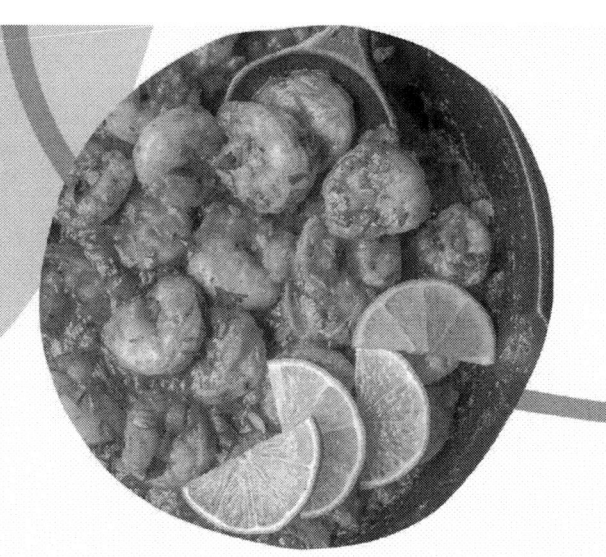

DIRECTIONS

1. Begin by rinsing the shrimp in cold running water. Use a kitchen paper towel to pat the shrimp dry and set it aside.
2. Take a shallow dish and fill it halfway with water. Place the skewers into the same to soak.
3. To prepare the marinade, take a small glass bowl and add in the tomato paste, oil, and water. Use a whisk to combine all the ingredients well. Also, add in the chili powder, oregano, and garlic. Whisk well.
4. Use a baking brush to coat both sides of the shrimp with the marinade and place them in the fridge for about half an hour.
5. Prepare the charcoal grill by lighting the fire. Take the grill rack and lightly grease it with cooking spray. Place the grill rack about 6 inches above the fire.
6. Insert the marinated shrimp into the skewers and place it onto the greased grill rack. Grill for 3 minutes; flip over and grill for another 3 minutes.
7. Transfer onto a serving platter and serve right away!

PORK MEDALLIONS IN FIVE SPICES

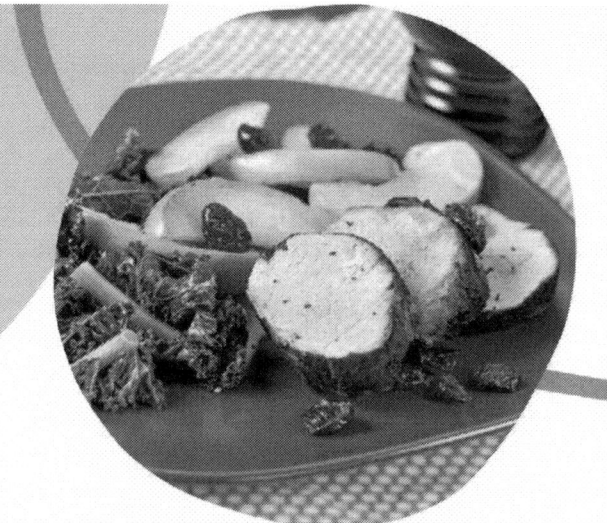

GENERAL INFO

Serving size: 1
Servings per recipe: 4
Calories: 413 calories per serving
Total time: 1 hour 20 minutes

INGREDIENTS

Canola oil – 1 tablespoon
Carrots (sliced) – 2 cups
Yellow onion (diced) – 1 cup
Fresh mushrooms – 1 cup
Fresh parsley (minced) – 2 tablespoons
Fancy wild rice (uncooked) – 1 cup
Walnuts (chopped) – 2 tablespoons
Black pepper (freshly ground) – 1 tablespoon
Chicken stock (no salt added) – 2 ½ cups
Chicken breasts (boneless and skinless) – 2
Red beets (diced) – 1 cup
Butternut squash (peel and dice) – 1 cup
Beet tops greens (chopped) – 2 cups
Balsamic vinegar – 1 tablespoon
Dried cranberries – 2 tablespoons

NUTRITION INFO

Protein – 26 g
Sodium – 184 mg
Carbohydrates – 57 g
Fat – 9 g

PORK MEDALLIONS IN FIVE SPICES

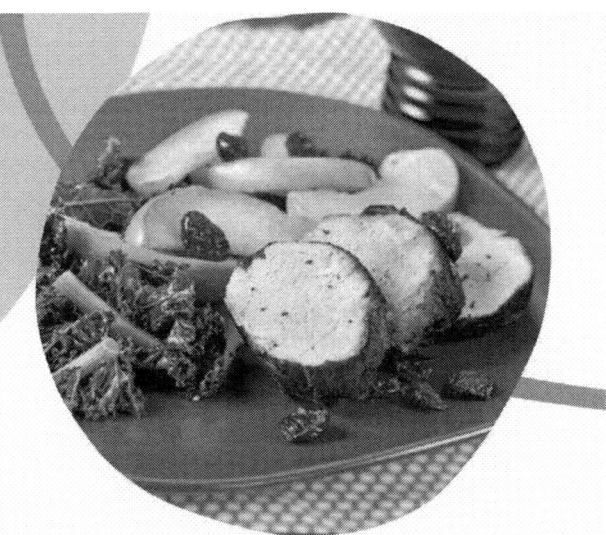

DIRECTIONS

1. Begin by heating a nonstick saucepan on a medium flame. Pour in ½ tablespoon of oil and let it heat through.
2. Once hot, toss in the carrots, mushrooms, parsley, and onion. Sauté for around 10 minutes or until they begin to caramelize.
3. Stir in the wild rice, chicken stock, walnuts, and black pepper; let it come to a boil and then reduce the flame. Cover the saucepan with a lid and cook for around 40 minutes.
4. While the rice is cooking, add the remaining half teaspoon of oil. Once the oil is hot, place the chicken breasts into the same and cook for around 3 minutes on each side.
5. Once done, remove the chicken onto a plate and set it aside.
6. Add the squash and beets to the pan; stir well and cook for about 20 minutes. The squash should be tender by now.
7. Add the prepared rice mixture, balsamic vinegar, chopped greens, and cranberries to the pan. Stir until well combined.
8. To serve, transfer into a serving bowl and top with chicken breasts.
9. Serve right away!

PUTTANESCA SERVED WITH BROWN RICE

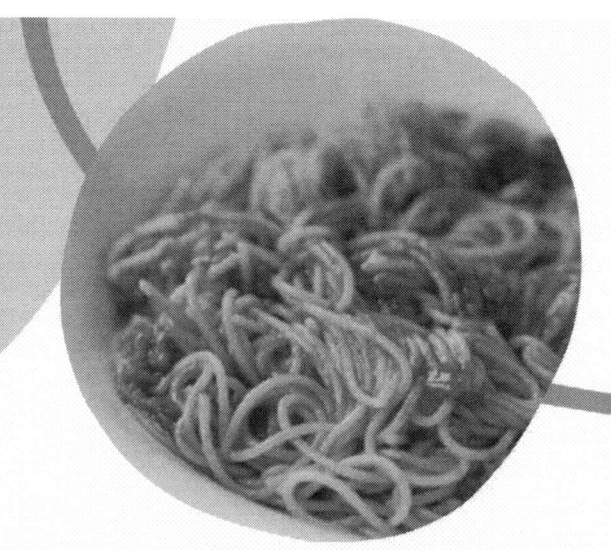

GENERAL INFO

Serving size: 2 cups
Servings per recipe: 4
Calories: 250 calories per serving
Total time: minutes

INGREDIENTS

Plum tomatoes (chopped) – 4 cups
Kalamata olives (sliced) – 4
Green olives (sliced) – 4
Capers (rinsed and drained) – 1 ½ tablespoons
Garlic (minced) – 1 tablespoon
Olive oil – 1 tablespoon
Fresh basil (chopped) – ¼ cup
Fresh parsley (minced) – 1 tablespoon
Red pepper flakes – ⅛ teaspoon
Brown rice (cooked) – 3 cups

NUTRITION INFO

Protein – 5 g
Sodium – 182 mg
Carbohydrates – 44 g
Fat – 6 g

PUTTANESCA SERVED WITH BROWN RICE

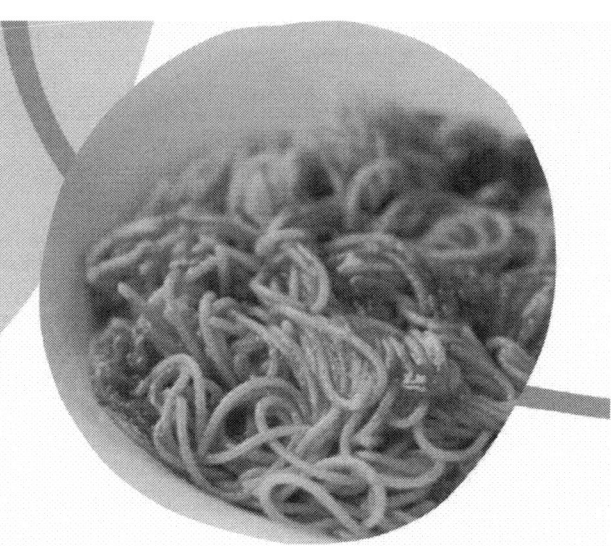

DIRECTIONS

1. Take a large glass mixing bowl and add in the chopped tomatoes, Kalamata olives, green olives, garlic, oil, and capers. Toss well.
2. Also, add in the parsley, red pepper flakes, and basil. Toss until all ingredients are well combined. Cover the glass bowl with a lid or cling film and let it sit for 30 minutes at room temperature. Give it a toss every 10 minutes.
3. To serve, take a plate and place the cooked rice into the same. Top with prepared puttanesca. Serve!

ROAST BALSAMIC CHICKEN

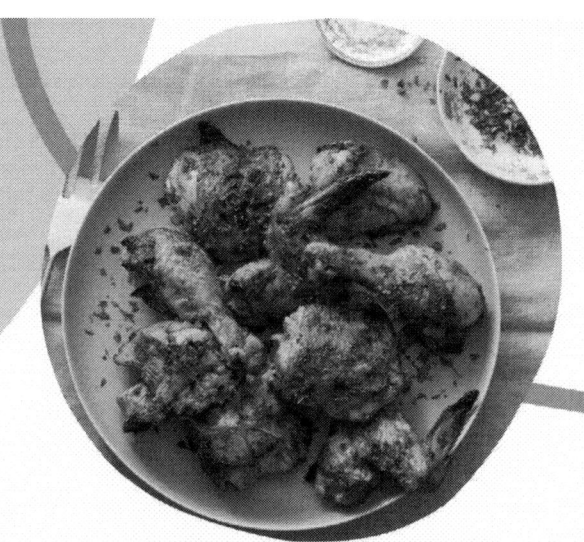

GENERAL INFO

Serving size: 1
Servings per recipe: 8
Calories: 301 calories per serving
Total time: 1 hour 40 minutes

INGREDIENTS

Whole chicken (skinned) – 1 (4 pounds)
Fresh rosemary (minced) – 1 tablespoon
Garlic (minced) – 1 clove
Olive oil – 1 tablespoon
Black pepper (freshly ground) – ⅛ teaspoon
Fresh rosemary – 8 sprigs
Balsamic vinegar – ½ cup
Brown sugar – 1 teaspoon

NUTRITION INFO

Protein – 43 g
Sodium – 131 mg
Carbohydrates – 3 g
Fat – 13 g

ROAST BALSAMIC CHICKEN

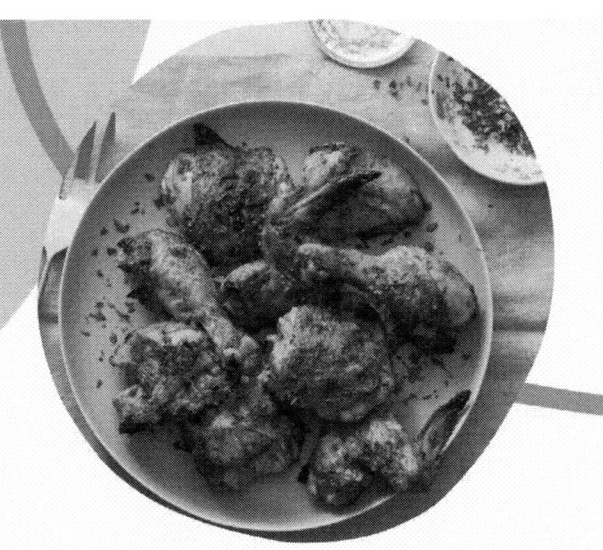

DIRECTIONS

1. Begin by preheating the oven by setting the temperature to 350 degrees Fahrenheit.
2. Take a small bowl and add in the minced garlic and minced rosemary. Mix well.
3. Place the chicken onto a plate and rub it with the oil and garlic mixture. Nicely sprinkle with freshly ground black pepper.
4. Take two sprigs of rosemary and put them into the chicken's cavity. Use butcher's twine to nicely truss the chicken.
5. Take a roasting pan and place the chicken into the same. Place the roasting pan into the preheated oven and roast for around 1 hour and 20 minutes. Baste the chicken after every 15-20 minutes to enhance the flavors.
6. Once the chicken has browned and the juices run clear, take the chicken out of the oven.
7. Transfer the chicken onto a serving platter and set aside.
8. Take a small nonstick saucepan and place it on a low flame. Add in the brown sugar along with the balsamic vinegar and let it heat until the sugar dissolves completely.
9. Carve the chicken and get rid of the skin. Pour the sugar and vinegar mixture over the chicken.
10. Finish by garnishing the chicken with rosemary and serve!

SOUTHWESTERN-STYLE VEGAN BOWL

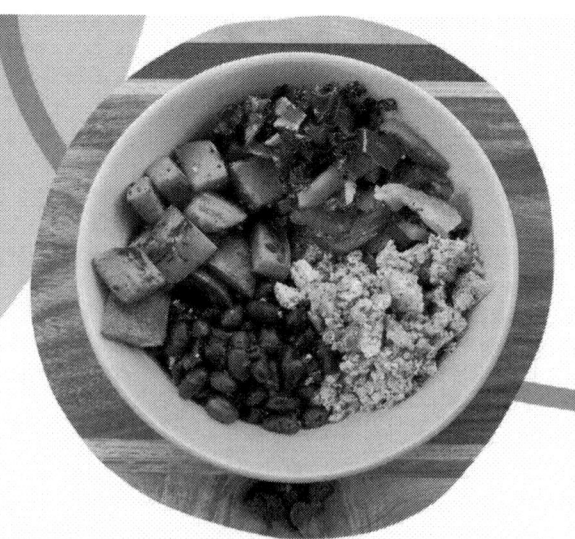

GENERAL INFO

Serving size: 2 cups
Servings per recipe: 6
Calories: 376 calories per serving
Total time: 1 hour 20 minutes

INGREDIENTS

Canola oil – 2 teaspoons
Red onion (chopped) – 1 cup
Green bell pepper (chopped) – 2 cups
Chili pepper (minced) – 1
Garlic (minced) – 2 cloves
Sweet potato (diced) – 1 cup
Tomato (chopped) – 1 cup
Brown rice – 1 cup
Green lentils – ½ cup
Red lentils – ½ cup
Ground cumin – 1 tablespoon
Pepper (freshly ground) – 1 tablespoon
Red wine vinegar – 1 tablespoon
Vegetable stock (no salt added) – 2 cups
Water – 2 cups
Kale (chopped) – 4 cups
Cooked black beans – 1 cup
Fresh cilantro (minced) – 2 tablespoons
Lime wedges – 4

NUTRITION INFO

Protein – 18 g
Sodium – 67 mg
Carbohydrates – 68 g
Fat – 4 g

SOUTHWESTERN-STYLE VEGAN BOWL

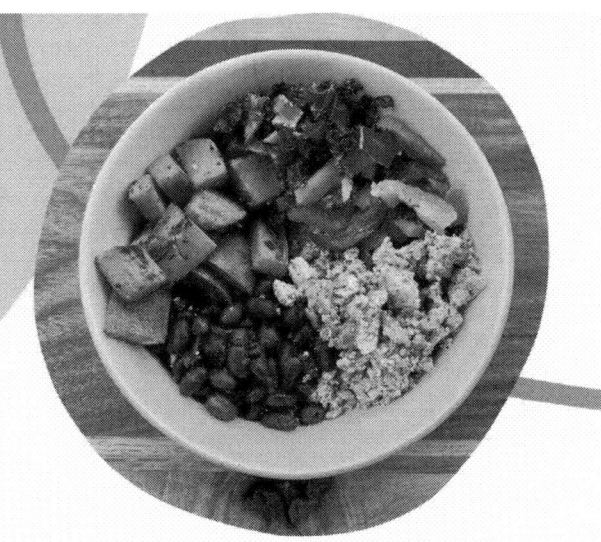

DIRECTIONS

1. Take a large saucepan and pour in the canola oil. Place the pan on a medium-high flame and let the oil heat through.
2. Toss in the onion, garlic, peppers, tomato, and sweet potato. Sauté for around 15 minutes or until the onions begin to appear translucent.
3. Now add the lentils, rice, spices, stock, water, and vinegar. Give the ingredients a nice stir and let it come to a boil.
4. Once you see the water bubbling, reduce the flame to low and cover with a lid. Cook on low for about 45 minutes. Stir every 15 minutes to prevent it from sticking to the bottom.
5. Once done, remove from the flame and add in the black beans, cilantro, and kale. Give it a nice stir.
6. Transfer into a serving bowl and top with lime wedges.
7. Enjoy!

VEGETARIAN TOFU CHILI

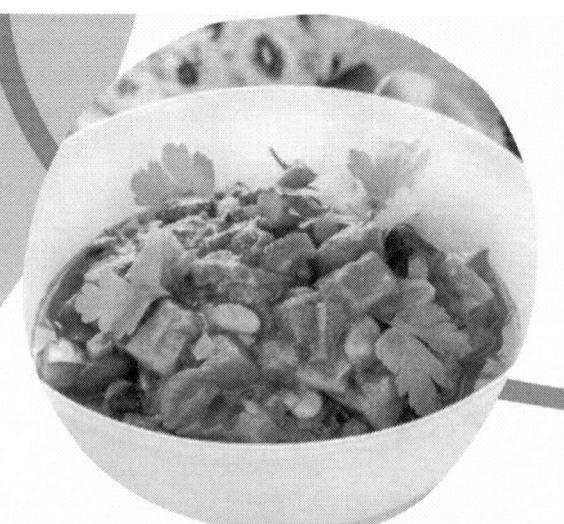

GENERAL INFO

Serving size: 2 cups
Servings per recipe: 4
Calories: 314 calories per serving
Total time: 45 minutes

INGREDIENTS

Olive oil – 1 tablespoon
Yellow onion (chopped) – 1 small
Tofu (extra-firm) – 12 ounces
Tomatoes (no added salt and diced) – 2 (14 ounces) cans
Kidney beans (no salt added) – 1 (14 ounces) can
Black beans (no salt added) – 1 (14 ounces) can
Chili powder – 3 tablespoons
Oregano – 1 tablespoon
Fresh cilantro (chopped) – 1 tablespoon

NUTRITION INFO

Protein – 19 g
Sodium – 364 mg
Carbohydrates – 46 g
Fat – 6 g

VEGETARIAN TOFU CHILI

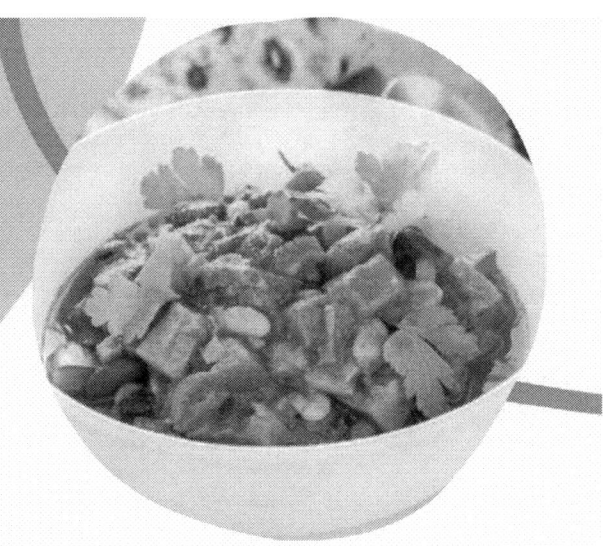

DIRECTIONS

1. Begin by cutting the tofu into small cubes measuring about ½ inch.
2. Now remove both the kidney beans and black beans from the can. Nicely rinse them and drain. Set aside.
3. Take a stockpot and place it on a medium flame. Pour the olive oil into the stockpot.
4. Once the oil is hot enough, toss in the onions and sauté for around 6 minutes. The onions should be translucent and not burnt.
5. Now add in the tomatoes, tofu, beans, oregano, and chili powder. Mix well and let it come to a boil.
6. Once the sauce begins to boil, reduce the flame and let the sauce cook for about 30 minutes.
7. Once done, remove from the flame and stir in the chopped cilantro. Mix well.
8. Transfer into a serving bowl and serve hot!

WHITE BROILED SEA BASS

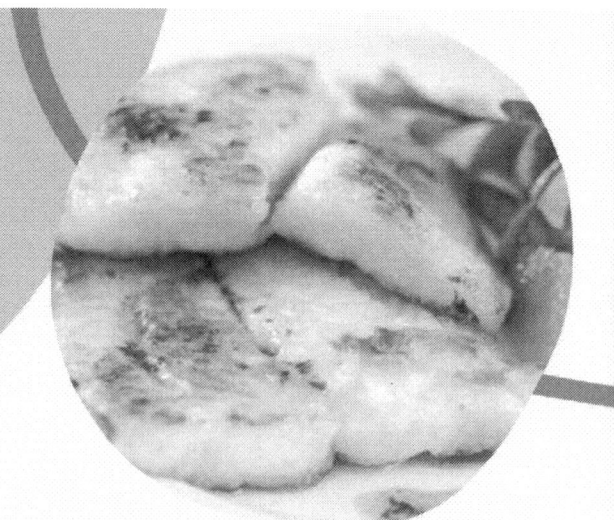

GENERAL INFO

Serving size: 1
Servings per recipe: 2
Calories: 102 calories per serving
Total time: 20 minutes

INGREDIENTS

White sea bass – 2 fillets
Lemon juice – 1 tablespoon
Garlic (minced) – 1 teaspoon
Herb seasoning blend (salt-free) – ¼ teaspoon
Black pepper (freshly ground) – as per taste

NUTRITION INFO

Protein – 21 g
Sodium – 77 mg
Carbohydrates – 0.5 g
Fat – 2 g

WHITE BROILED SEA BASS

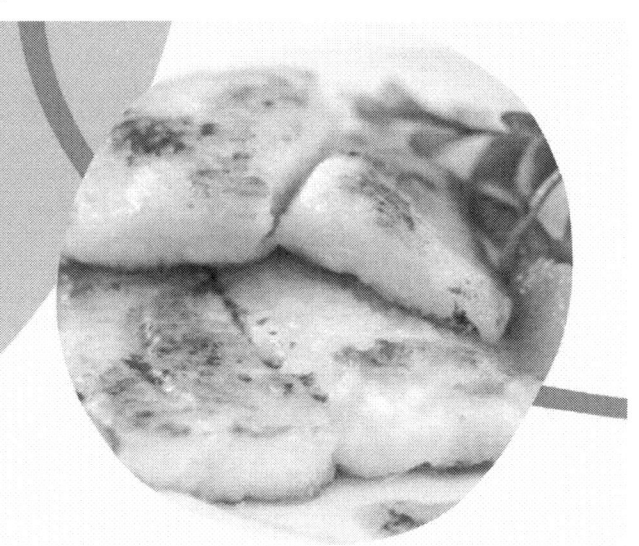

DIRECTIONS

1. Begin by heating the broiler and placing the rack at least 4 inches away from the heat.
2. Take a baking sheet and grease it generously with nonstick cooking spray.
3. Place the sea bass fillets onto the baking sheet and season them with lemon juice, herbed seasoning, pepper, and garlic.
4. Place the baking sheet into the oven and broil for around 10 minutes.
5. Serve right away!

An Appeal from the Publisher

Hello wonderful reader!

We hope you are enjoying this book.

We wanted to let you know that you have made an impact on many lives by reading this book.

Just to give you a brief introduction: We are a small publishing company with a team of 8 writers and 2 editors.

Most of our employees come from financially weaker section and our company is the only means they support their families. This is our way of giving back to the society.

We don't have the giant advertising budgets that many other publishers and businesses do online.

So, one way that you can really support our mission and our business is by leaving us a review on this book.

For a small company like us, getting reviews (especially on Amazon) means we can submit our books for advertising.

This means we can actually sell a few copies from time to time and make a bigger impact on the society as a whole. So, every review means a lot to us.

We can't THANK YOU enough for this!

THANK YOU

Made in the USA
Middletown, DE
05 June 2021